Nutritious and Delicious

who knew healthy could taste so good?

revision 3

5-2012

MARIA EMMERICH

CONTENTS

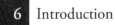

INTRODUCTION

HOW TO BALANCE OUR WEIGHT, MOODS AND LIFE!

So often we focus on calorie reduction for weight loss because we are told metabolism comes down to calories in, calories out. This is really only one piece of the puzzle. If you are eating 500 calories of carbohydrates at a meal you are going to be storing a lot more fat. However, if those 500 calories are a combination of protein, carbohydrates, and fat, you could actually burn fat!

Sadly, the food industry has been adding empty calories to traditional foods. In the early 1970s, food manufacturers started adding a cheap substance to foods...high fructose corn syrup. Corn is cheap and abundant, and thanks to government subsidies, American's desire for sweets has increased tenfold. Over the past fifteen years, our food industry has increased products filled with carbohydrates such as adding unneeded sweeteners to marinara sauce, baby formula, ketchup, yogurts, and chicken breasts. Yes, I said chicken breasts. McDonald's grilled chicken breast ingredients list is: *Chicken breast filets with rib meat, water, seasoning (salt, sugar, food starch-modified, maltodextrin, spices, dextrose, autolyzed yeast extract, hydrolyzed [corn gluten, soy, wheat gluten] proteins, garlic powder, paprika, chicken fat, chicken broth, natural flavors (plant and animal source), caramel color, polysorbate 80, xanthan gum, onion powder, extractives of paprika), modified potato starch, and sodium phosphates.* WHAT a joke! **Here's a terrifying statistic: the average piece of chicken's protein content has dropped by a third since 1971!**

We're relentlessly told that carbohydrates are the good guys of nutrition, and that, if we eat large amounts of them, the world will be a better place. The "food pyramid" tells us, there will be no heart disease and no obesity. With these words of wisdom, Americans are gobbling cereals, breads and pastas as if they were preparing for a marathon, trying desperately to reach that 75 to 85% of total calories advocated by the high-carb fanatics.

A recent Harvard University study found that people who had the highest saturated fat intake also had the *least* plaque buildup on their artery walls. The *American Journal of Clinical Nutrition* described the findings as an "American Paradox." In a Stanford University study that made recent headlines, women on the "fatty" Atkins diet ended up with the healthiest cholesterol levels and the best blood pressure readings, compared to those on other diets, notably the famous high-carb low-fat diet.

Since the 1970s, American men have decreased their saturated fat intake by 14% and increased their carbohydrate intake by 23% --yet rates of obesity and heart disease are increasing. The more carbs you eat, the higher your insulin levels climb, which signals your liver to produce saturated fat. If you go on a healthy-carb diet, your insulin levels drop, and so does production of saturated fat.

This is creating a terrible paradox: people are eating less fat and getting fatter! Overeating carbohydrate foods can prevent a higher percentage of fats from being used for energy, and lead to a decrease in endurance and an increase in fat storage. There is an alarming conclusion discovered: a high- carbohydrate, low-fat diet may be dangerous to your health.

Eating fat does not make you fat. It's your body's response to excess carbohydrates in your diet that makes you gain weight. Your body has a limited capacity to store excess carbohydrates, but it can easily convert those excess carbohydrates into excess body fat.

It's hard to lose weight by simply restricting calories. Eating less and losing excess body fat do not necessarily go hand in hand. Low-calorie, high-carbohydrate diets generate a series of biochemical signals in your body that will take you out of the balance, making it more difficult to access stored body fat for energy. As a result, you will reach a weight-loss plateau, beyond which you simply can't lose any more weight.

People on restrictive diets get tired of feeling hungry and deprived. Diets based on calorie limits and choice restriction usually fails. People are unsatisfied, go off their diets, put the weight back on as increased body fat, and then feel like a failure for not having enough will power or discipline.

The success to weight loss has little to do with discipline. You need the proper information to make powerful changes. People need to focus on WHAT to eat rather than HOW MUCH. Eating a diet of low carbohydrate meals, you can eat enough to feel satisfied and still wind up losing fat without obsessively counting calories or fat grams.

Sadly, many people don't really know what a carbohydrate is. Most people will say carbohydrates are sweets and pasta. They often think a vegetable or fruit as a food type all its own; a food that they can eat in unlimited amounts without gaining weight. This may come as a surprise, but sweets and pasta, vegetables and fruits are all carbohydrates. Carbohydrates are merely different forms of simple sugars linked together in polymers. We all need a certain amount of carbohydrates in our diet. The body requires a continual intake of carbohydrates to feed the brain, which uses glucose as its primary energy source. In fact, the brain is a virtual glucose hog, gobbling more than two thirds of your carbohydrate stores in the bloodstream while you are at rest. To feed this glucose hog, the body constantly takes carbohydrates and converts them to glucose.

The process is a bit more in-depth than that. Any carbohydrates not immediately used by the body will be stored in the form of glycogen. The body has two storage sites for glycogen: the muscles and the liver. The glycogen stored in the muscles is inaccessible to the brain. Only the glycogen stored in the liver can be sent back to the bloodstream so as to maintain adequate blood sugar levels for proper brain function. **A normal blood sugar is 1 TEASPOON of sugar in our bloodstream! The average person consumes more than 65 teaspoons of GRANULATED sugar every day…on top of the excess carbohydrates!**

The liver's capacity to store carbohydrates in the form of glycogen is very limited and can be easily depleted within ten to twelve hours. So the liver's glycogen reserves must be maintained on a continual basis. That's why we eat carbohydrates. The trick is to choose the right ones to sustain our blood sugar levels for the optimal time.

What happens when you eat too many carbohydrates? No matter where the carbohydrates are being stored, liver or the muscles, the total storage capacity of the body for carbohydrate is really quite limited. **In the liver, where carbohydrates are accessible for glucose conversion, you can store only about 60-90 grams.** This is equivalent to about two cups of cooked pasta or three bananas.

Once the levels in the liver are filled with glycogen, excess carbohydrates have just one fate: to be converted into fat and stored. Even though carbohydrates are fat-free, excess carbohydrates end up as excess fat. But that's not the worst of it. Any meal or snack high in carbohydrates will generate a rapid rise in blood glucose. To adjust for this rapid rise, the pancreas secretes the hormone insulin into the bloodstream. Insulin then lowers the levels of blood glucose. **The problem is that insulin is mainly a storage hormone; it works to put aside excess carbohydrate calories in the form of fat in case of a future food shortage. The insulin that's stimulated by too many carbohydrates assertively promotes the accumulation of body fat. To recap, when we eat too much carbohydrate, we are sending a hormonal message, through insulin, to the body that states: "Store as fat".** They also tell it not to release any stored fat. When this happens, you can't use your own stored body fat for energy. So the excess carbohydrates in your diet not only make you fat, they make sure you stay fat.

After you eat carbohydrates your pancreas releases insulin and your blood sugar increases. Insulin makes sure your cells receive some blood sugar necessary for life, and increases glycogen storage. But, it also tells your body to use more carbohydrate, and less fat, as fuel. Insulin also converts almost half of your carbohydrate intake to fat for storage in-case of an energy emergency. If you want to burn fat for energy, the insulin response must be decreased. Eating refined sugars release a lot of insulin, allowing less stored fat to be burned.

High insulin levels also suppress two important hormones: growth hormone and glucagon. Growth hormone is used for muscle development and building new muscle mass. Glucagon promotes the burning of fat and sugar. Eating a high carbohydrate meal also stimulates hunger. As blood sugar increases, insulin rises with an immediate drop in blood sugar. This results in hunger, often only a couple of hours after the meal. Cravings, usually for sweets, are frequently part of this cycle, leading you to snack on more carbohydrates. Not eating makes you feel ravenous, shaky, moody and ready to "crash." This cycle causes you to never get rid of that extra stored fat, and causes a decrease in energy.

Does this sound like you? The best suggestion for anyone wanting to utilize more fats is to moderate the insulin response by limiting the intake of refined sugars, and keeping all other carbohydrate intake to about 30% of the diet. Proteins and fats don't produce much insulin. Eating protein and fat while eating carbohydrates can slow the increase in blood sugars significantly. Having peanut butter with an apple is a great option.

Insulin responses are different in everybody. However, refined foods increase insulin reactions. The main reason is that refined carbohydrates lack the natural fiber which helps minimize the insulin response. Eating natural fiber with carbohydrates can reduce the blood sugar reactions described above. Low-fat diets cause quicker digestion and absorption of carbohydrates in the form of sugar. By always adding some fats to your diet, you will slow down digestion and absorption, and the insulin reaction won't be so extreme. Decreasing refined carbohydrates and increasing fats will help bring your body back into balance. By moderating carbohydrate intake you can increase your fat burning as an optimal fuel source.

We evolved for hundreds of thousands of years from the so-called "cave man's diet," which consisted of meat and vegetables. With the onset of modern civilization, our physiology suddenly was asked to digest and metabolize larger amounts of starch and refined sugars. We are unable to utilize the amount of carbohydrates we eat; therefore, certain symptoms develop.

OVERCONSUMPTION OF REFINED CARBOHYDRATES:

1. **Fatigue:** The most common feature of Insulin Resistance is that it makes people exhausted. Some are tired only in the morning or afternoon; others are wiped all day.

2. **Brain fog**: Insulin Resistance is often mental. Not being able to concentrate is the most evident symptom. Poor memory, failing or poor grades in school are often a side effect of Insulin Resistance. Are you sending your kids off to school with a bowl of cereal and skim milk??? Not a good idea.

3. **Low blood sugar**. Feeling jittery and moody is common in Insulin Resistance, with an immediate relief once food is eaten. Dizziness is also caused by low blood sugar, as is the craving for sweets.

4. **Intestinal bloating**. Most intestinal gas is produced from too many carbohydrates. People with Insulin Resistance who eat carbohydrates suffer from gas, lots of it. Antacids or other remedies for symptomatic relief are not very successful in dealing with the problem.

5. **Tired After Meals**. Being sleepy after meals containing more than 20% or 30% carbohydrates is a main side-effect. This is typically a pasta meal, or even a meat meal which includes bread or potatoes and a sweet dessert.

6. **Increased fat storage and weight**. In males, a large abdomen is the more evident and earliest sign of Insulin Resistance. In females, it is stored in the hips and thighs.

7. **Increased triglycerides**. Even normal weight individuals may have stores of fat in their arteries as a result of Insulin Resistance.

8. **Increased blood pressure**. Doctors now recognize that most people with hypertension have too much insulin and are Insulin Resistant. There is often a direct relationship between the level of insulin and the level of blood pressure: as insulin levels increase, so does blood pressure.

9. **Depression**. Carbohydrates are a natural "downer," depressing the brain; it is not uncommon to see many depressed persons also having Insulin Resistance. Carbohydrates change the brain chemistry. Carbohydrates produce depressing or a 'tired' feeling. On the flip side, protein is a brain stimulant, picking you up mentally.

10. **Alcoholism**: Insulin Resistance is also prevalent in people addicted to alcohol, caffeine, cigarettes or other drugs. Often, the alcohol is the secondary problem, with Insulin Resistance being the primary one. Alcohol becomes sugar in our bodies. This is why recovering alcoholics

often overeat sweets, which causes a relapse…we never kicked the true addiction…sugar!

HOW TO BECOME BALANCED

1. **Protein**. Know how much protein your body needs. Don't consume more protein than your body requires, but more importantly, never consume less. Finding your balance can be tricky. On average, protein requirements range from 60 grams per day for a sedentary obese individual to as much as 200 grams per day for a lean heavily exercising athlete. You should have protein in EVERY meal to help balance hormone levels.

2. **Carbohydrates**. You should also choose your carbohydrates wisely. If you are insulin resistant, have high blood pressure, high cholesterol, high blood pressure or are overweight then you need to specifically restrict your carbohydrates to low starch vegetables, low sugar fruits and whole grains filled with fiber. Starchy-refined carbohydrates cause inflammation in our body which aggravates existing health issues. If you find yourself hungry and craving sugar two to three hours after a meal, you probably ate too many carbohydrates in the previous meal. If you have a problem with hunger or carbohydrate cravings, look at what you ate for a clue to the problem. Decrease the amount of carbohydrates and increase the amount of protein.

3. **Fat.** Olive oil and fish are great choices. Healthy fats help balance out hormone levels and decrease inflammation. Stick with natural fats, such as butter and cheese. Think about eating as natural as possible. "American" cheese is anything but natural! Fat also is essential to decrease the fat storing hormone, insulin.

4. **Water**. Try to drink around 64 ounces of water per day. Hydrated cells balance hormone levels. Caffeine tends to increase insulin levels, so go easy on the coffee.

5. **Exercise**. Exercise is very helpful for balancing insulin levels. Try to get 30 to 60 minutes of walking most days a week.

Eggs for breakfast! What about my cholesterol levels?
The most common misperception about cholesterol is that there's something unhealthy about cholesterol. Cholesterol is one of the body's repair substances: Its elevated presence in your system tells you that your body is trying to heal something; such as inflammation; which is the true source of the problem. Most Americans consume 200-300mg of cholesterol, but our body needs around 1000mg a day, so our body will produce the rest...no matter what. Our body makes extra because cholesterol is essential for hormone function, particularly the ones the body needs during stressful times. When people use statin drugs to reduce their cholesterol, instead of focusing on ridding the foods causing the inflammation (processed, fried foods) it causes muscles to deteriorate; which we know slows metabolism.

FOOD SUBSTITUTIONS FOR HIGH CARB ITEMS

Many everyday food ingredients are very high in sugar and bad carbs. These tables show the various substitutions I use in my recipes. Use this chart to understand the healthier alternatives and why I have selected various ingredients for my recipes.

Milk Substitutions (Per Cup)					
FOOD	Rate	Carbs	Sugars	Fiber	Calories
Skim Milk	Bad	13	13	0	91
Unsweetened Almond Milk	Best	2	0	1	40
Coconut Milk	Best	1	0	0	50

Rice Substitutions (Per Cup)					
FOOD	Rate	Carbs	Sugars	Fiber	Calories
White Rice	Bad	53	0	0	242
Brown Rice	Bad	46	0	4	218
Quinoa	Bad	39	0	5	222
Wild Rice	Bad	35	1.2	3	166
Cauliflower Rice	Best	3	1	1	28

Pasta Substitutions (Per Cup)					
FOOD	Rate	Carbs	Sugars	Fiber	Calories
White Pasta	Bad	43	0	5	246
Spaghetti Squash	OK	10	4	2	42
Bean Sprouts	Best	6	4	2	31
Artichoke Hearts	Best	6	0	4	40
Cabbage	Best	5	3	2	22
Eggplant noodles	Best	5	2	3	20
Zucchini	Best	4	2	1	20
Miracle Noodles	Best	0	0	0	0

Potato Substitutions (Per Cup)					
FOOD	Rate	Carbs	Sugars	Fiber	Calories
Potato	Bad	28	2	4	116
Sweet Potato	Bad	27	6	4	114
Celeriac(celery root)	OK	14	2	3	66
Rutabaga	OK	11	8	4	50
Turnips	Best	8	5	2	36
Jicama	Best	11	2	6	46
Daikon Radish	Best	2	0	1	30
Cauliflower	Best	3	1	1	28
Radishes	Best	4	2	2	19

Snack/Dips (Per 6 oz. container)					
FOOD	Rate	Carbs	Sugars	Fiber	Calories
Yoplait Yogurt	Bad	35	28	0	175
Plain Yogurt	Bad	17	10	1	120
Sour Cream	Best	7	0	0	364
Cottage Cheese	Best	9	6	0	120

Corn Substitution (Per Cup)					
FOOD	Rate	Carbs	Sugars	Fiber	Calories
Corn	Bad	30	5	4	132
Baby Corn	Best	4	0	4	36

Fruit Substitutions (Per Cup)					
FOOD	Rate	Carbs	Sugars	Fiber	Calories
Dried Fruit (Cranberry)	Bad	96	75	3	390
Banana	Bad	51	27.5	5.9	200
Grapes	Bad	29	24.8	1.4	110
Apple	Bad	21	17	4	95
Raspberries	OK	14	5.4	8	64
Strawberries	OK	11.7	2.9	6	46
Jicama (apple texture)	Best	11	0	6	46
Chayote (apple texture)	Best	5.1	2.4	2.2	22

Flour Substitutions (Per Cup)					
FOOD	Rate	Carbs	Sugars	Fiber	Calories
Rice Flour (GLUTEN-free foods)	Bad	127	0.2	3.8	578
White Flour	Bad	100	0	4	496
Wheat Flour	Bad	87	0	14	407
Oat Flour	Bad	78	0	12	480
Almond Flour	Best	24	4	12	640
Coconut Flour	Best	80	0	48	480
Peanut Flour	Best	21	4	9	196
Flaxseed meal	Best	32	0	32	480

Bread Substitutions (Per Slice)					
FOOD	Rate	Carbs	Sugars	Fiber	Calories
White	Bad	22	3	3	110
Whole Wheat	Bad	20	3	3	100
Ezekiel	Bad	15	0	3	80
Trader Joe's Sprouted Wheat	Bad	7	0	3	60
My Flaxseed Bread	Best	5	0	5	185
My Protein Bread	Best	Trace	0	0	60

Condiment Substitutions (Per 1/4 cup)					
FOOD	Rate	Carbs	Sugars	Fiber	Calories
Famous Dave's BBQ Sauce	Bad	32	30	0	120
Ketchup	Bad	16	16	0	60
Reduced Sugar Heinz Ketchup	OK	4	4	0	20
Salsa (not fruit/ corn/bean based)	Best	5	4	1	20
French dressing	Bad	16	12	1	260
Raspberry Vinaigrette	Bad	12	12	0	160
Ranch Dressing	Best	2	2	0	280
Ranch Dressing (50-50 with Beef Stock)	Best	1	1	0	140

Cereal Substitutions (Per Cup)					
FOOD	Rate	Carbs	Sugars	Fiber	Calories
Kashi Go Lean	Bad	30	10	6	148
Fiber One	Bad	50	0	28	120
Instant Oatmeal (apple cinnamon)	Bad	26	12	3	130
Homemade "faux" oatmeal	Best	7	0	5	140

Food Substitutions For High Carb Items

OTHER (Per 4 TBS)					
FOOD	Rate	Carbs	Sugars	Fiber	Calories
Jelly (4 TBS)	Bad	48	48	0	400
Nature's Hollow Jelly	Best	8*	0	0	80
Pancake Syrup	Bad	40	40	0	240
Nature's Hollow Syrup	Best	28*	2	0	76
Honey (4 TBS)	Bad	70	70	0	240
Nature's Hollow Honey	Best	32*	0	0	80

* Non-effective carbohydrate (Sugar Alcohol)

Cracker Substitutions (Per 25 grams)					
FOOD	Rate	Carbs	Sugars	Fiber	Calories
Wheat Thins	Bad	16	1	3	112
Dr. In the Kitchen Flackers	Best	8	0	7	110
Homemade Almond Flour Crackers	Best	3	0	1	114

SWEETENER CONVERSION

1 cup erythritol and 1 tsp stevia = 1 cup ZSweet or Truvia

1 cup erythritol and 1 tsp stevia = 1 cup Swerve

1 cup erythritol and 1 tsp stevia = 1 cup Xylitol

1 cup erythritol and 1 tsp stevia = 1 cup Just Like Sugar

1 cup erythritol and 1 tsp stevia = 1 cup Organic Zero and 1 tsp stevia

HARD TO FIND INGREDIENTS AND TOOLS:

For all the special ingredients and tools I use go to my Amazon aStore at:

astore.amazon.com/marisnutran05-20

I have created an AMAZON.COM store where you can find all the healthy ingredients that are difficult to find in the grocery store (and if you do find them, they are often very expensive). I have done some detective work and found the lowest prices on www.amazon.com for all of the products I use and love. Everything from food, pantry items, kitchen tools, supplements and skin products are in the aStore. I rarely waste time in the grocery store because I find everything online for a way better price!

You can also continue shopping for other products on Amazon after you are finished with "healthified" shopping. Just click the "Proceed to Checkout". It then asks you if you want to add these to your Amazon cart (at the main Amazon site). Just click "Continue" and now you can add whatever else you want from Amazon all in the same cart! I always choose at least one thing from my Amazon Store before moving onto other items I need for the family, those items will also help pay for the blog without any extra cost; I just get a small commission for bringing your business to Amazon.com. Happy Shopping and THANK YOU for all your support!!!

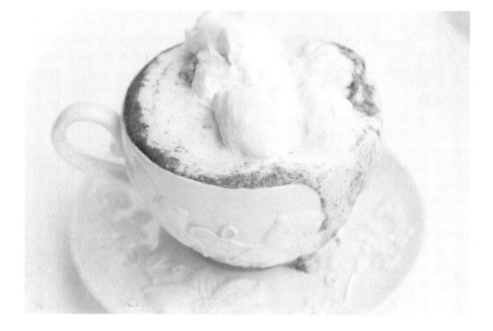

TRIPLE HOT CHOCOLATE

I always enjoyed a little warm drink around the campfire, but I had a hard time finding a replacement for the good-old packages of hot chocolate mixes that have trans-fat in them. NESTLE HOT COCOA INGREDIENTS: SUGAR, CORN SYRUP SOLIDS, VEGETABLE OIL **(PARTIALLY HYDROGENATED COCONUT OR PALM KERNEL AND HYDROGENATED SOYBEAN)**, DAIRY PRODUCT SOLIDS (FROM MILK), COCOA PROCESSED WITH ALKALI, AND LESS THAN 2% OF SALT, CELLULOSE GUM, SODIUM CASEINATE, POTASSIUM PHOSPHATE, SODIUM CITRATE, SODIUM ALUMINOSILICATE, MONO- AND DIGLYCERIDES, GUAR GUM, ARTIFICIAL FLAVORS, SUCRALOSE.

"Healthified" Hot Chocolate:

1 chocolate hazelnut tea bag

Few drops of chocolate stevia

1 cup unsweetened chocolate almond milk

If you wanted to make it "a quadruple" hot chocolate, you could also add a TBS of unsweetened cocoa powder!

NUTRITIONAL COMPARISON:

Swiss Miss "Sugar Free" Hot Chocolate = 60 calories, 10 carbs, 7 sugar (made with WATER!)

"Healthified" Hot Chocolate = 40 calories, 1 carb, 0 sugar

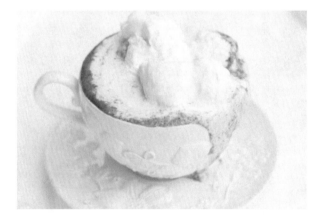

IRISH CREAM

1 1/2 cups Unsweetened Vanilla/Chocolate Almond Milk
2 TBS cocoa powder (or 1 oz. 100% chocolate bar)
2 1/2 tsp instant coffee granules
2 TBS Jay Robb vanilla whey
1/4 tsp almond extract
1/4 tsp vanilla extract
3 drops Stevia Glycerite
Optional: 2/3 cup Irish Whiskey

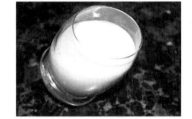

Place all ingredients in a saucepan. Warm until chocolate is melted. Remove from heat and place in your blender, and run until smooth and well-blended. Makes 2 servings.

NUTRITIONAL COMPARISON Per 1 cup Serving:
REAL Irish Cream = 2,150 calories, 45.34 carbs, 0 fiber
"Healthified" Irish Cream = 110 calories, 6 carbs, 3 fiber

PUMPKIN LATTE

1.5 cups vanilla almond milk
1 tsp pumpkin pie spice (or a dash of: cinnamon, nutmeg, ginger and cloves)
4 TBS canned pumpkin
1 tsp pure vanilla
Sweetener to taste
1 shot of espresso (or 1/4 cup strong coffee)

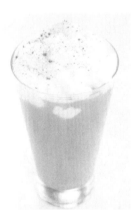

In a saucepan, warm the almond milk, spice, pumpkin, vanilla and sweetener until hot. Place the espresso in a cup. Slowly add the almond milk into the espresso and enjoy!

NUTRITIONAL COMPARISON (per 16 ounces):
Starbucks Pumpkin Latte = 288 calories, 54 carbs, 0 fiber, 50g sugar!
"Healthified" Latte = 67.5 calories, 3.75 carbs, 2g fiber, 0 sugar

STIR FRY SAUCE

1 cup wheat free Tamari (or soy sauce)

2 tsp rice wine vinegar

2 tsp toasted sesame oil

1 tsp hot red pepper flakes

2 drops Stevia Glycerite

2 tsp fresh grated fresh ginger

1 large clove minced garlic

1 cup chicken stock

1-1/2 tsp guar gum (thickener)

Combine tamari sauce, vinegar, oil, pepper flakes, ginger, garlic and stevia in a small bowl until well combined. In a separate small bowl whisk together chicken stock and guar gum; let sit until thickened. Slowly add the broth mixture into the tamari mixture. Store in fridge for up to one week.

Nutritional Information for the WHOLE batch = 195 calories, 6 carbs, 2 fiber

ALL-NATURAL ALMOND MILK

1 1/2 cups of raw almonds
4 cups of filtered or spring water

Blend 1 1/2 cups of raw almonds that have been soaked overnight in 4 cups of water. Blend with pure vanilla extract if you like your milk with a hint of sweetness. Strain once to remove almond granules. The result is delicious, creamy milk that is free of harmful vegetable oil, and sweeteners. It can be stored safely for 3-4 days in the refrigerator.

Nutritional Information (per cup) = 40 calories, 2 carbs, 1 fiber

ICED CHAI LATTE

1 Chai Tea Bag
16 oz. vanilla almond milk (or coconut)
3 or 4 drops Stevia Glycerite

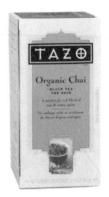

In a saucepan, warm the almond milk, nutmeg and sweetener until hot. Place the tea bag in a tea cup. Slowly add the almond milk into the cup and let steep for 3 minutes. Enjoy!

NUTRITIONAL COMPARISON:
Starbuck's Chai Latte = 240 calories, 47 carbs, 1 fiber

"Healthified" Chai Latte = 80 Calories, 4 carbs, 2 fiber, 0 sugar

EGGNOG

1 eggnog tea bag
1 cup vanilla almond milk
1/4 tsp nutmeg
1 drop of Stevia Glycerite

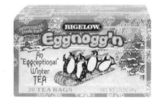

In a saucepan, warm the almond milk, nutmeg and sweetener until hot. Place the tea bag in a tea cup. Slowly add the almond milk into the cup and let steep for 3 minutes. Enjoy!

NUTRITIONAL COMPARISON (per cup):
Traditional eggnog = 343 calories, 34.4 carbs, 0 fiber
"Healthified" eggnog = 42 calories, 2 carbs, 1 fiber

A TRUE EGGNOG

4 eggs, separated
4 drops Stevia Glycerite
1 pint almond milk
3 oz. bourbon (optional)
1 tsp freshly grated nutmeg

Beat the egg yolks until they lighten in color. Gradually add the stevia and set aside. In a medium saucepan, over high heat, combine the almond milk and nutmeg and bring just to a boil, stirring occasionally. Remove from the heat and gradually temper the hot mixture into the egg and stevia mixture. Then return everything to the pot and cook until the mixture reaches 160 degrees F. Remove from the heat, stir in the bourbon, pour into a medium mixing bowl, and set in the refrigerator to chill. In a medium mixing bowl, beat the egg whites until stiff peaks form. Whisk the egg whites into the chilled mixture.

NUTRITIONAL COMPARISON (per 1 cup)
Traditional Eggnog = 343 calories, 34 carbs, trace fiber
"Healthified" Eggnog = 110 calories, 3 carbs, 2 fiber (*without Bourbon)

GRAVY

4 egg whites
1/4 cup wheat free Tamari
sauce (soy sauce)
1/8 tsp dried thyme or
poultry spice
1/4 cup chicken broth
2 TBS sour cream
2 drops Stevia Glycerite
Celtic sea salt & pepper to
taste

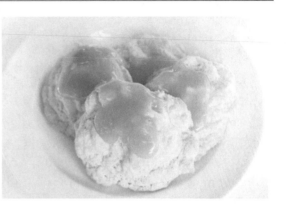

On medium heat cook egg whites mixed with tamari sauce, broth & spices until the eggs are cooked and a bit lumpy. Pour into a blender, add sour cream and stevia and blend for 1 minute until smooth. Makes 16 servings.

NUTRITIONAL COMPARISON:
Traditional Gravy = 20 calories, 4 carbs, 0 fiber, 1g protein
"Healthified" Gravy = 11 Calories, 0.4 carbs, 0 fiber, 1g protein

GINGER SAUCE

1 TBS peeled and minced ginger
1/2 cup expeller pressed Olive Oil
1/4 cup scallions, white and green parts combined, cut into 1/4 inch pieces
Celtic sea salt to taste
2 TBS wheat free tamari (or soy sauce)
1 tsp sesame oil

To make the sauce, stir together in a bowl. The mixture should be quite strong; you can add more ginger, scallions, or salt if you like.

FAT FLUSH SEASONING:

1/3 cup dried parsley

1/4 cup ground cumin

2 TBS onion powder

2 TBS garlic powder

2 tsp ground coriander

1 tsp minced lemon zest

1/4 tsp cayenne pepper

1/2 packet stevia

Combine all ingredients and store in a container away from stove. Use on eggs, meat, seafood, anything really!

TASTY HOMEMADE MAYO

1 cup light olive oil (or walnut or sweet almond oil)

1 egg yolk

Juice of 1 lemon, or vinegar

A pinch of Celtic sea salt (and pepper, if desired)

Chicken broth to thin the mayonnaise

Separate the eggs in your recipe. Reserve the whites for other recipes. Egg yolks contain a natural emulsifier, lecithin, which helps thicken sauces and bind ingredients. Lemon juice or vinegar adds acidity to the mayonnaise. It also helps flavor the mayonnaise, which, incidentally, has quite a low pH, so is inhospitable for bacteria. Mayonnaise is rarely the culprit in food-borne illness cases: it's much more likely to be the potatoes or pasta in the picnic salads causing problems! For each cup of mayonnaise, add between 1 and 2 tablespoons of fresh lemon juice or vinegar, depending upon your tastes. Combine the egg and acid in the bowl, whisking to mix. You can make mayonnaise in a food processor or by hand, with a mixing bowl and whisk. The key for either method is to add oil very slowly, in a steady stream, while the processor is running or you're whisking vigorously. If the mayonnaise starts looking too thick, add enough broth to thin it to the consistency you desire. Add about a teaspoon of broth at a time. When the oil is all mixed in, the mayonnaise should be thick and fluffy. Adjust the seasoning with the salt and pepper and more acid, if desired. Store in the refrigerator and use within five days. Makes 1 cup. **Nutritional Information** (per TBS) = 78 calories, 0.1 carbs, 0 fiber, 0.2 protein

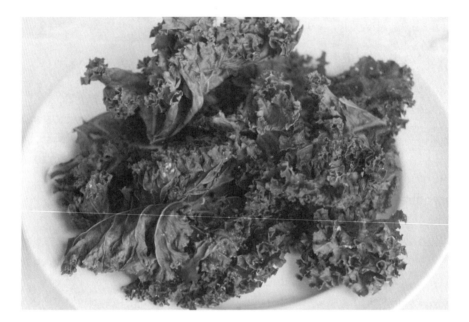

TORTILLA CHIPS

2 medium sized turnips/zucchini (about 2 cups), shredded
2 cups sharp cheddar cheese, freshly shredded
2 eggs

Preheat the oven to 425 degrees F. Shred the turnips and cheese. Mix all ingredients together. Grease a cookie sheet. Place 6 round circles on the cookie sheet (not too close, they will spread). Bake for 15 minutes. Flip circles, cut with a pizza cutter into chip shapes, and bake for another 5 minutes or until crisp and golden brown. Leave them in a closed oven for another 20 minutes. They will continue to crisp up.. Makes 8 servings.

NUTRITIONAL COMPARISON (per serving):
Traditional Tortilla Chips = 138 calories, 18.6 carbs, 1.2 fiber
"Healthified" Tortilla Chips = 138 calories, 2.4 carbs, 0.6 fiber

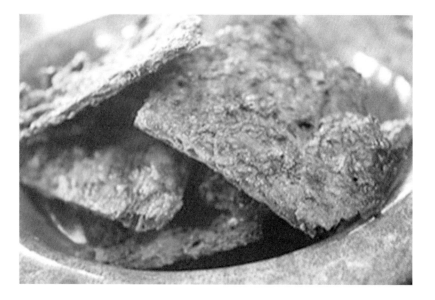

CRAB RANGOON

"Wrappers" AKA "Puffs":

3 eggs, separated

1/2 tsp cream of tartar

3 oz. Sour Cream or cream cheese

1/2 cup unflavored whey protein

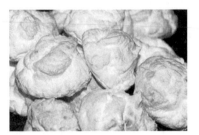

Preheat oven to 375 degrees F. Separate the eggs and reserve the yolks for another recipe (crème brule anyone?). In a large bowl, whip egg whites and cream of tartar until VERY stiff. Then add the whey. Using a spatula, gradually fold the sour cream into the egg white mixture, being careful not to break down the whites. Place round balls of dough onto a GREASED baking sheet (or a mini muffin tin works great). Bake at 375 degrees F for 10 minutes, then turn oven off. Keep oven shut, and leave the puffs in there for another 5 minutes or until cool. Makes 24 puffs. Nutritional info (per puff): 21 calories, trace carbs, 0 fiber, 2.3g protein

Filling:

1 clove garlic, minced

1 (8 oz.) package cream cheese

1 (6 oz.) can crabmeat, drained and flaked

2 green onions with tops, thinly sliced

1 tsp fresh ginger, finely grated

1/2 tsp wheat-free organic Tamari (soy sauce)

Combine garlic, cream cheese, crab, green onions, ginger, and Tamari sauce in a bowl. Fill into puffs. To prevent puffs from getting soggy, fill the day you plan on eating. Makes 8 servings.

NUTRITIONAL COMPARISON (per serving)

Traditional Crab Rangoon = 261 calories, 29.2 carbs, 1 fiber, 11.2 protein

"Healthified" Crab Rangoon = 177.5 calories, 2.1 carbs, 1 fiber, 16.8g protein

SAVORY PARTY PUFFS

Puffs:

3 eggs, separated
1/2 tsp cream of tartar
3 oz. Sour Cream or cream cheese
1/2 cup Parmesan cheese, grated

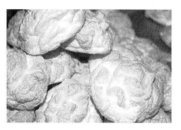

Preheat oven to 375 degrees F. Separate the
eggs and reserve the yolks for another recipe (crème brule anyone?). In a
large bowl, whip egg whites and cream of tartar until VERY stiff. Then
add the Parmesan cheese. Using a spatula, gradually fold the sour cream
into the egg white mixture, being careful not to break down the whites.
Place round balls of dough onto a GREASED baking sheet (or a mini
muffin tin works great). Bake at 375 degrees F for 10 minutes, then turn
oven off. Keep oven shut, and leave the puffs in there for another 5
minutes or until cool. Makes 24 puffs.

NUTRITIONAL COMPARISON (per puff):
Traditional Puff = 76 calories, 6.9 carbs, trace fiber, 1.9 protein
"Healthified" Puff = 26 calories, trace carbs, 0 fiber, 2.3g protein

FILLING:

2 packages (8 oz. each) cream cheese, softened
2 packages (2 oz. each) thinly sliced deli corned beef, chopped
1/2 cup homemade mayonnaise
1/4 cup sour cream
2 TBS minced chives
2 TBS diced onion
1 tsp spicy brown or horseradish mustard
1/8 tsp garlic powder
10 small pimiento-stuffed olives, chopped

In a large bowl, combine the first eight filling ingredients. Stir in olives.
Split puffs; add filling. Refrigerate.

SCOTCH EGGS

Coconut oil or Ghee for frying
4 eggs
2 pounds lamb or pork sausage
8 TBS (2 TBS per egg) coconut flour, seasoned with spices
2 eggs, beaten

Preheat oven to 350 degrees F. Heat oil in a pan to 375 degrees F. Place eggs in saucepan and cover with water. Bring to boil. Cover, remove from heat, and let eggs sit in hot water for 10 to 12 minutes. Remove from hot water, cool and peel. Flatten the sausage and make a patty to surround each egg. Coat the sausage with beaten egg. Roll in coconut flour to cover evenly. Fry until golden brown. Place on a cookie sheet and bake in the preheated oven for 10 minutes.

NUTRITIONAL COMPARISON:
"Traditional" Scotch Egg = 300 calories, 16 carbs, 0 fiber
"Healthified" Scotch Egg = 230 calories, 9 carbs, 4 fiber.

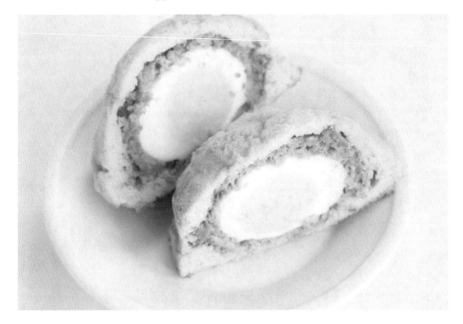

GREEK AVOCADO DIP

1 (8 oz.) container cottage cheese
2 avocados - peeled, pitted, and mashed
1 clove garlic, minced
2 TBS lime juice
1 Roma (plum) tomato, seeded and diced
1/4 cup crumbled feta cheese
Celtic Sea Salt and Pepper to taste

Mash together the avocado, garlic, and lime juice in a bowl until nearly smooth. Place in a food processor and add cottage cheese and blend until very smooth. Fold in the diced tomato and feta cheese. Add salt and pepper to taste. Serves 6: That's A LOT of DIP!

Nutritional Information (per serving) = 150 Calories, 7.7 Carbs, 4.7 fiber, 6.2 protein

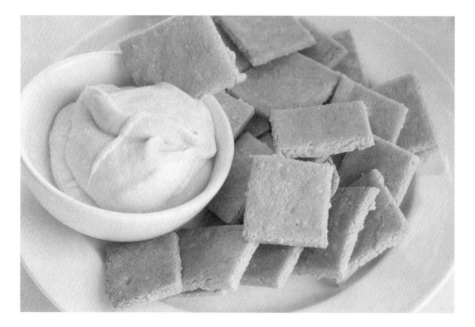

PRIMAL POPPERS

1 8-oz. package cream cheese
15 jalapeno peppers
1 package nitrate free bacon

De-seed peppers. Using a knife, split the pepper on one side from the bottom to the top. Gut out all of the seeds and fibrous innards. Stuff the pepper full of cream cheese. Wrap the pepper in a slice of bacon. Arrange on a baking tray. "Pop" in the oven at 425 degrees F for 15 minutes. Serve with salsa or guacamole or just serve plain. Enjoy!

NUTRITIONAL COMPARISON:
Traditional Poppers = 220 calories, 18 carbs, trace fiber, 4 protein
"Healthified" Poppers = 150 calories, 1.7 carbs, trace fiber, 5.3 protein

KOREAN BARBECUE BITES

1 skirt steak
1 cucumber
2 TBS wheat free tamari sauce (soy sauce)
1/2 tsp Stevia Glycerite
1 tsp sesame oil
1 tsp grated ginger
2 cloves garlic, minced

Cut skirt steak into 30 strips, and slice a cumber with a vegetable peeler into ribbons. Thread together on skewers, and marinate 10 minutes in a mixture of 2 tablespoons soy sauce, 1/2 tsp Stevia Glycerite, 1 teaspoon each sesame oil and grated fresh ginger, and 2 minced garlic cloves. Grill on each side 1 1/2 minutes. Makes 30 servings.

Nutritional Information (per serving) = 20 calories, 1 g Fat, 2 g protein, 1g carb, 0g fiber

RUEBEN FRITTERS

Coconut oil or Expeller pressed Safflower oil, for frying
1 can (8.8-oz., drained weight) sauerkraut
4 oz. corned beef, chopped into pieces
4 oz. swiss cheese, shredded
5 TBS chopped chives, divided
2 tsp minced garlic, divided
2 eggs, separated
3 TBS heavy cream
1 cup Blanched almond flour
2 tsp baking powder
3/4 tsp salt, divided
1 tsp Essence, plus more for seasoning, recipe follows
1 avocado, diced
2 TBS olive oil mayonnaise
2 TBS lime juice
2 TBS minced green onions
1 jalapeno pepper, seeded and minced (optional)
1 tsp hot sauce
1/4 tsp cayenne pepper

Heat a deep-fryer or a Dutch oven or deep cast iron skillet filled halfway with oil to 360 degrees F. Place the sauerkraut onto a paper towel and let drain thoroughly, then place it into a bowl and add the meat and cheese.

In a small mixing bowl combine 3 TBS of the chives, 1 tsp of the garlic, egg yolks and heavy cream and whisk well to combine. Add the egg mixture to the sauerkraut, corned beef and swiss, and blend gently to combine. In a separate bowl, stir together the almond flour, baking powder, 1/4 tsp of the salt and Essence. Stir the flour mixture into the hearts of palm mixture until just combined. In a clean mixing bowl beat the egg whites until medium to stiff peaks form. Fold the whites into the sauerkraut mixture very gently and let sit for 5 minutes before frying. While the fritter batter is resting, make the dipping sauce by combining the avocado, mayonnaise, lime juice, green onions, jalapeno, jalapeno hot sauce, cayenne pepper, remaining 2 TBS of chives, remaining teaspoon of garlic, and remaining 1/2 teaspoon of salt in the bowl of a food processor and process until thoroughly smooth, stopping to wipe down the sides of the bowl, if necessary. Taste and adjust seasoning. Set aside until ready to serve the fritters. Drop the batter by 1 1/2 tablespoonfuls into the hot oil and fry the fritters, in batches if necessary, until golden brown, turning, 2 to 3 minutes per side. Remove fritters using a slotted spoon and transfer to paper towel-lined plate to drain. Season with sea salt to taste and serve immediately, with the avocado dipping sauce.

B-L-TEASERS

30 small butter lettuce leaves
15 grape tomatoes
30 pieces pancetta
60 pieces pearl mozzarella
Pesto Sauce
Fresh Basil leaves

Top 30 small butter lettuce leaves with halved grape tomatoes, cooked pancetta, pearl mozzarella, a drizzle of pesto, and fresh basil leaves (bottom right).

Nutritional Information (per serving) = 24 calories, 1g Carb, 0g fiber, 2g Fat, 1g Protein

1/2 cup unflavored whey (Jay Robb)
3/4 cup blanched almond flour
1/4 tsp baking soda
1/4 tsp Celtic sea salt
1/4 cup butter
2 TBS water (to hold dough together)
1 additional large egg (to brush on pastry)

Filling: Fill with crab, pesto, cheese, ground nuts or olives, or any combination thereof. Brush the tops with additional egg wash and sprinkle with poppy or sesame seeds if desired. Preheat the oven to 350 degrees F. In a medium bowl, stir together the

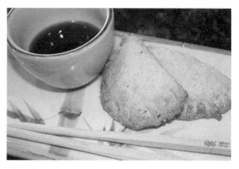

whey, almond flour, baking soda and salt. Cut in the butter using a pastry blender or your fingers until the butter lumps are smaller than peas. Stir in the water to form a stiff dough. On parchment paper, place 16 balls of dough a few inches apart. Shape with hands into rectangle shapes (This recipe will make a batch of 16 2 1/4" x 3" rectangles or ovals.). Beat the additional egg and brush it over the entire surface of the rectangles. Even the "insides" of the tart; the egg is to help glue the lid on. Place a heaping tablespoon of filling into the center of each rectangle, keeping a bare 1/8-inch perimeter around it. Fold the other side over and using your fingertips, press firmly around the pocket of filling, sealing the dough well on all sides. Press the tines of a fork all around the edge of the rectangle. Repeat with remaining tarts. You could either freeze the filled tarts or bake them at this time. Gently place the tarts on a lightly greased or parchment-lined baking sheet. Prick the top of each tart multiple times with a fork; you want to make sure steam can escape, or the tarts will become fluffy pillows instead of flat toaster pastries (my mistake number 1). Bake for 10-12 minutes in the preheated oven, until edges are lightly browned. Cool in oven to crisp up. Serve with Ginger Sauce (pg.

31). Makes 16 servings.

Nutritional Information (per serving) = 62 calories, 1 carb, trace fiber

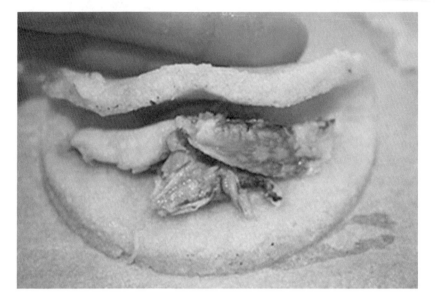

STUFFED PEPPAS

30 mini peppers
30 tsp goat cheese
Toasted Pine nuts

Fill each of 30 peppadew peppers with 1 teaspoon softened herbed goat cheese; top with toasted pine nuts. Makes 30 servings

Nutritional Information (per serving) = 43 calories, 2g Fat, 1g Protein, 4g Carbs, 0.5g fiber

PARTY APARAGUS

8 cups water
3 TBS Celtic Sea salt
1 pound asparagus, thick spears work best

Bring the water to a boil in a pot. When the water comes to a boil, add the salt. While the water comes to a boil, fill another pan with ice, then cold water. Have this ready before the asparagus goes into the boiling water, you want it to be really cold. Meanwhile, peel the skins off the asparagus, about half-way up. Snap off the woody ends. Drop all the asparagus at once into the pan and let cook for 4-8 minutes or until done, it depends on how thick the spears are. Once they're done, remove from heat and immediately drop into the ice water. Leave them in the water just long enough to cool down (you don't want them soggy), then immediately transfer onto paper towels to drain and dry, tapping the top sides too. These can be made several hours in advance.

AIOLI:
2 garlic cloves, chopped small
1 egg yolk
2 tsp lemon juice
1/2 tsp Dijon mustard
7 TBS extra-virgin olive oil
Salt & pepper to taste

Whisk together the garlic, yolk, lemon juice and mustard -- alternatively do a whiz or two in a small food processor (there's not enough volume for a big food processor). Slowly drizzle in the olive oil while whisking or processing, being sure to incorporate what's been added before adding more. Makes 14 servings.

Nutritional Information (per serving) = 75 Calories, 0 carb, 0 fiber

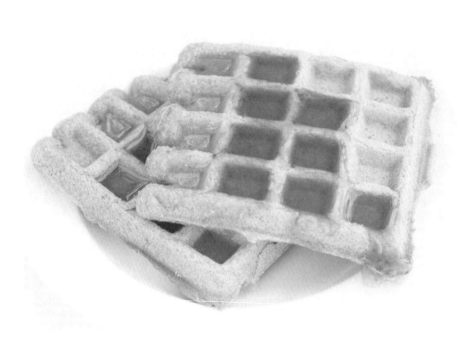

CHOCOLATE CAKE DONUTS

1/2 cup blanched almond flour
3 eggs, separated
1/4 cup Erythritol and 1 tsp Stevia Glycerite
1/4 tsp Celtic sea salt
1/4 tsp baking soda
1 tsp vanilla
1/4 tsp cinnamon
2 TBS cocoa powder
4 TBS coconut oil or
butter
Frosting:
1 ChocoPerfection Bar
1 TBS unsweetened
almond milk (or cream)

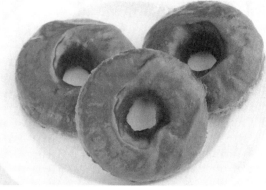

Whip the egg whites until stiff peaks form. Combine the yolks, sweetener, oil/butter and whisk until well-blended. Combine all the dry ingredients, blend well. Gently fold the wet ingredients into the whipped whites and then slowly fold in the dry mixture, and fold until well blended. Fill the donut pan 3/4 of the way full. Bake for 15 minutes at 350 degrees F, or until a toothpick comes out clean.

Meanwhile: Melt the chocolate bar (in 10 second intervals in microwave) and add in whipping cream. Once the donut is cooled, dip in melted ChocoPerfection Chocolate Bar! Makes 8 donuts.

NUTRITIONAL COMPARISON:
Traditional Cake Donut = 290 calories, 33 carbs, 1 fiber
"Healthified" Donut = 123 calories, 3.75 carbs, 2.5 fiber

MINI FILLED DONUTS

1/2 cup vanilla whey (Jay Robb)
2 tsp baking powder
1/8 tsp Celtic sea salt
4 TBS vanilla almond milk
1 egg
1/8 cup Erythritol and a drop
of Stevia Glycerite
Coconut oil or Ghee
For Filling:
Nature's Hollow
Jelly (optional)
For Topping:
3 TBS Erythritol
Pinch cinnamon

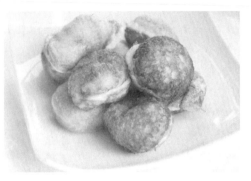

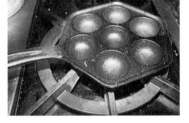

Mix topping ingredients and set aside.
Whisk dry ingredients together. Whisk
egg with other wet ingredients, add to
dry ingredients, and whisk to combine well. Fill a donut skillet, cast-iron
pan, or dutch oven with oil and heat. When oil reaches around 350 to
360 degrees F, drop batter into the oil. The batter will spread and puff
up. When the underside browns, flip. In another 30 to 45 seconds, it will
be ready to remove. Be sure to enjoy them ASAP, as they will lose their
crisp if they sit too long. Cut a hole with a knife through the middle and
fill with jelly. I placed the jelly into a small ziplock and cut a small hole
into the corner. I then squeezed the jelly into the hole. Sprinkle with
Erythritol and cinnamon. Serves 12.

Nutritional Information (per serving) = 26 calories before frying (then it
depends on the oil absorption), less than 1 gram of effective carbs

REECE'S PEANUT BUTTER DONUTS

2 cups peanut flour
1/2 cup Erythritol and 1/2 tsp Stevia Glycerite
3 1/2 tsp aluminum free baking powder
1 tsp Celtic sea salt
1/8 tsp baking soda
1 1/4 cups vanilla almond milk
1 tsp vanilla
3 large eggs

Preheat oven to 350 degrees F. Line cupcake pans with paper liners or you may also grease cupcake pans with butter. Combine all ingredients in a large mixing bowl. Mix at low speed for 30 seconds while scraping bowl. Mix at high speed for 3 minutes, scraping bowl every minute. Spoon batter into greased donut pan until they are 2/3 full. Bake for 20 to 25 minutes or until toothpick inserted in center comes out clean. Cool 10 minutes in pans then move to wire rack to cool completely. Frost your peanut butter donuts with chocolate icing.

CHOCOLATE ICING:
6 TBS unsweetened cocoa powder
1/4 cup butter
1/4 cup Erythritol (powdered)
1/4 cup vanilla almond milk
1/2 tsp vanilla extract

To make the frosting, make erythritol into a powder in a food processor. Melt together the 6 tablespoons of cocoa and butter; set aside to cool. In a medium bowl, blend together the sweetener, almond milk and 1/2 teaspoon vanilla. Stir in the cocoa mixture. Spread over cooled donuts and enjoy!

<u>OR EASY ICING</u>:
1 ChocoPerfection Bar
1 TBS unsweetened almond milk

Melt the chocolate, mix with almond milk. Then spread over donuts.
Makes 12 donuts.

NUTRITIONAL COMPARISON:
Dunkin' Donuts Cake Donut = 380 calories, 36 carbs, 2g fiber, 4g
protein
"Healthified" Donut = 170 calories, 4.3 carbs, 2g fiber, 7g protein

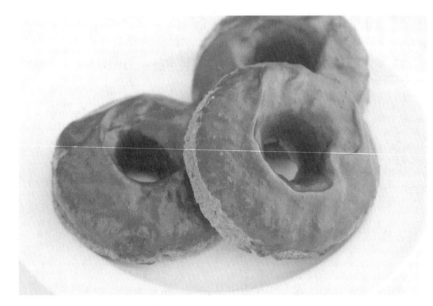

PUMPKIN DONUTS WITH PUMPKIN GLAZE

1 1/2 cups blanched almond flour
1/4 tsp Celtic sea salt
1/2 tsp baking soda
1 tsp ground cinnamon
1/2 tsp ground nutmeg
1/4 tsp ground ginger
1/8 tsp ground cloves
2 TBS Butter or Coconut Oil
1/3 cup Erythritol and 1/2 tsp Stevia Glycerite
3 large eggs
1 cup fresh OR canned pumpkin

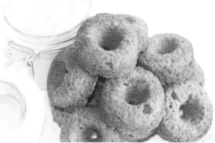

In a mixing bowl combine almond flour, baking soda, salt, and spices. Mix butter, sweetener, eggs and pumpkin until smooth. Stir wet ingredients into dry. Grease donut pan. Spoon batter into the pan. Bake at 325 degrees F for 30-40 minutes. Cool and top with pumpkin glaze!

Pumpkin Glaze:
8 oz. cream cheese
1/2 cup pureed pumpkin
1/2 cup vanilla almond milk
1 tsp vanilla
1 tsp cinnamon
1 tsp pumpkin pie spice
3 to 4 drops Stevia Glycerite to taste
Combine all the ingredients in a medium bowl and beat until smooth. Let sit for 4 hours or overnight...it will thicken up. Serves 6.

NUTRITIONAL COMPARISON (per donut):
Krispy Kreme Pumpkin Spice Donut = 340 calories, 42 carbs, 1 fiber
"Healthified" Pumpkin Spice Donut = 198 calories, 7.7 carbs, 2.8 fiber

EGGNOG FRENCH TOAST

EGGNOG BREAD:

4 eggs, separated
1 cup vanilla whey (Jay Robb)
4 drops of Stevia Glycerite
1/2 cup unsweetened almond milk
1 tsp nutmeg

Separate the eggs. Place the egg whites in the bowl of a stand mixer and beat to stiff peaks. Slowly add the whey. Set aside. In a large bowl, beat the egg yolks until they lighten in color. Add the stevia and continue to beat for 2 minutes. Add the almond milk and nutmeg and stir to combine. Slowly stir the egg whites into the mixture. Grease a bread loaf pan. Place the mixture into the pan. Bake at 350 degrees F for 50 minutes. Cool completely and cut into 12 large pieces.

Nutritional Information (per slice) = 43 calories, 0.6 carbs, trace fiber

For FRENCH TOAST:

2 eggs
1/2 cup vanilla almond milk
1 tsp vanilla
1 tsp nutmeg
1 loaf Eggnog Bread

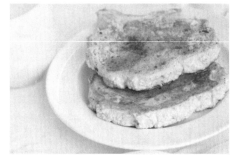

Place first 4 ingredients in a bowl. Dip the slices of eggnog bread into the egg mixture, fry on both sides until golden brown. Serve with Nature's Hollow Maple Syrup.

SYRUP NUTRITIONAL COMPARISON (1/4 cup syrup):
Regular Pancake Syrup = 240 calories, 40 carbs, 40 sugar
Nature's Hollow Syrup = 76 calories, 2 effective carbs
Walden Farms Syrup = 0 calories, 0 carbs, 0 sugar

CREAM CHEESE DANISH

Pastry portion:
3 large eggs, separated (reserving 1/2 yolk for filling)
1/4 tsp. cream of tartar
1/4 cup Erythritol and 1/4 tsp Stevia Glycerite
1 tsp cinnamon
3 TBS sour cream
1/2 cup Vanilla Whey Protein

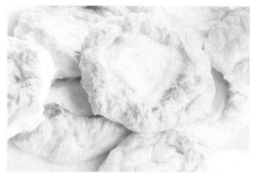

Filling:
4 oz. cream cheese, softened
1/2 egg yolk (from above)
1/4 cup Erythritol and 1/4 tsp Stevia Glycerite
1/4 tsp vanilla
Optional: 1/4 tsp lemon, almond, orange, or raspberry extract

Pastry directions: Separate eggs, putting the whites in a large bowl and the yolks in a medium bowl. Take 1/2 yolk out and put it in a little dish to reserve for filling. With your electric beater, whip whites and cream of tartar until very stiff, then add the whey protein. Add sour cream, cinnamon, sweetener to the yolks and beat well until smooth. Gently fold yolk mixture into the whites, using a big spatula, being careful to get it all blended well. Then spray a cookie sheet or muffin top pan (the best way), and plop 6 equal mounds of batter to make 6 Danish. Make an indent on each mound and fill with filling. To make filling: Soften cream cheese and add the 1/2 egg yolk, sweetener, extract, and flavoring. Fill the pastries. Bake about 25-35 minutes at 300 degrees F until golden brown. Remove, cool and enjoy. Makes 4 servings.

NUTRITIONAL COMPARISON:
Starbuck's Danish = 440 calories and 61 carbs!!!
"Healthified" Danish = 168 calories and 3 carbs

COCONUT FLOUR CAKE DONUTS

1/2 cup coconut flour

1/4 tsp Celtic sea salt

1/4 tsp baking soda

6 eggs

1/2 cup Erythritol and 1 tsp Stevia Glycerite

1 TBS vanilla

1/2 cup coconut oil or butter

Preheat oven to 350 degrees F. Blend all the dry ingredients together in a bowl. Blend in all the wet ingredients into the dry ingredients. Mix until well-blended. Fill donut pan circles about 2/3 of the way full with batter. Bake for about 20 minutes, or until a toothpick comes out clean.

Toasted coconut topping: Toast some unsweetened coconut flakes for about 5 minutes at 300 degrees F. Dip each donut in sugar free pancake syrup and then in the toasted coconut. Makes 8 donuts.

NUTRITIONAL COMPARISON (per donut):

Traditional Cake Donut = 192 calories, 23 carbs, trace fiber

"Healthified" Cake Donut = 182 calories, 5.7 carbs, 3 fiber

DRY CEREAL

2 TBS sliced almonds
2 TBS ground almonds
2 TBS organic golden flax meal
1 TBS vanilla whey protein
Pinch Salt
2 TBS water

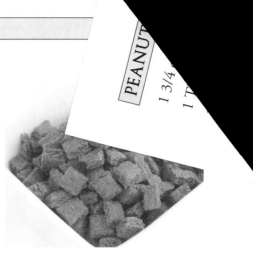

In small cereal bowl, combine sliced
almonds, ground almonds, flax meal,
vanilla whey protein, and salt. Stir in
water. Spray dinner plate with nonstick cooking spray. Spread mixture
out in large circle on plate. Microwave 3 minutes on high. Break into
irregular, small pieces. Serve with unsweetened vanilla almond milk and
stevia to taste. Makes 1 serving.

Nutritional Information = 214.0 calories, 2.1 g carbs, 1.9g fiber, 12.0 g
protein, 16.6 g fat

PROTEIN WAFFLES

1 cup almond flour
1 cup vanilla whey protein
1/2 tsp Celtic sea salt
1 TBS aluminum free baking
powder
1 1/2 cup vanilla almond milk
2 eggs
4 TBS butter or coconut oil

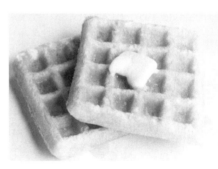

Preheat waffle iron to high. Combine the dry ingredients in a bowl.
Combine the wet ingredients in another bowl. Stir wet into dry. Makes 6
double waffles, 12 singles.
Nutritional information (per single waffle) = 121 calories, 2.5 carbs, 1.1
fiber

cup peanut flour

BS baking powder

1 tsp Stevia Glycerite

1/4 tsp Celtic sea salt

2 eggs

1 cup vanilla unsweetened almond milk

1/2 cup softened butter

Preheat waffle iron. In a medium sized bowl, mix the dry ingredients together. In a separate bowl, mix the wet ingredients together. Slowly mix the dry ingredients into the wet and mix until smooth. Make sure the iron is hot and add the batter onto the greased waffle iron. Close the iron and cook according to directions (3-5 minutes) or until crisp. These tasted great by themselves or with a little butter melted on top! Makes 6 Double Waffles (or 12 singles).

Nutritional Information (per single waffle) = 104 calories, 3.1 carbs, 1.5 fiber, 5.25 protein

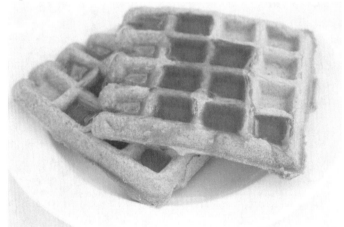

PUMPKIN PANCAKES

1/4 cup cottage cheese

2 eggs

1/4 cup pumpkin

1/4 tsp cinnamon

1 tsp vanilla

1/2 tsp baking powder

2 TBS flaxseed

2 drops Stevia Glycerite

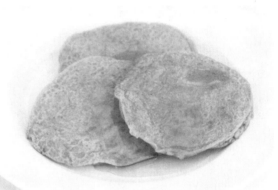

Preheat skillet. Beat eggs
with electric mixer on high for 1 minute to make them light and fluffy.
In a food processor, blend the cottage cheese until very smooth, then add
to the eggs. Add all the other ingredients. Pour batter onto skillet, fry
until golden brown. Serve with Nature's Hollow syrup. Makes 4
servings. Whole Recipe = 321 calories, 11.9 carbs, 6.6 fiber

NUTRITIONAL COMPARISON (per serving):
Traditional Pancakes = 149 calories, 28 carbs, 1 fiber, 4g protein
"Healthified" Pancakes = 80 calories, 2.9 carbs, 1.6 fiber, 9g protein

NUTRITIONAL COMPARISON (1/4 cup syrup):
Regular Pancake Syrup: 240 calories, 40 carbs, 40 sugar
Nature's Hollow Syrup: 76 calories, 2 effective carbs
Walden Farms Syrup: 0 calories, 0 carbs, 0 sugar

PROTEIN PANCAKES

1/2 cup cottage cheese
2 eggs
1/2 cup Jay Robb vanilla whey protein
2 TBS vanilla unsweetened almond milk
2 tsp baking powder
1 drop Stevia Glycerite

Place all ingredients in a food processor and blend until smooth. Let sit for 5 minutes (the baking powder will "fluff" up the batter). Heat a skillet and cook! I can take out this entire recipe without any guilt! But it serves 4. Just be careful with what you smear on top! You can easily get up to 500 calories and a sugar coma with maple syrup. Makes 4 servings. ENTIRE RECIPE: 369 Calories, 7 carbs, 52g protein.

NUTRITIONAL COMPARISON:
Traditional Pancakes = 149 calories, 28 carbs, 1 fiber, 4g protein
"Healthified" Pancakes = 90 calories, 1.75 carbs, trace fiber, 13g protein

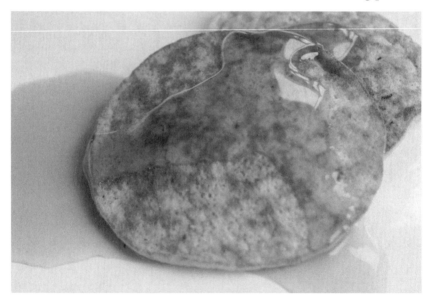

PEANUT FLOUR PANCAKES

1 3/4 cup peanut flour
1 TBS aluminum free baking powder
4 drops Stevia Glycerite
1/4 tsp Celtic sea salt
2 eggs
1 cup vanilla unsweetened almond milk
1/2 cup softened butter

Preheat skillet. In a medium sized bowl, mix the dry ingredients together. In a separate bowl, mix the wet ingredients together. Slowly mix the dry ingredients into the wet and mix until smooth. Makes 24 small pancakes.

Nutritional Information (per pancake) =58 calories, 1.6g carbs, 0.7g fiber, 3g protein

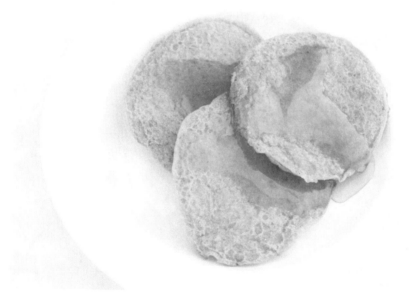

 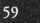

DUTCH PANCAKES

Dutch pancakes are a fluffy pancake baked in the oven. My tip is to make the batter the night before and place it in the oven when you get out of bed. By the time you are done showering and getting the kids up, the pancakes will be nice and warm, fresh out of the oven!

Butter or coconut oil (to grease pan)
1/2 tsp Celtic sea salt
1/4 cup coconut flour
1 tsp baking soda
1 tsp baking powder
6 eggs
1 cup coconut milk or vanilla almond milk
Toppings: Nature's Hollow maple syrup, Nature's Hollow honey,

Preheat oven to 425 degrees F. Grease the bottom and sides of a 9 x 13 glass baking pan with butter or coconut oil. Whisk all the dry ingredients together and add in the eggs and coconut milk until batter is well smooth. Pour into greased pan. Bake for about 20-25 minutes until puffed and cooked all the way through. Serve immediately. Makes 4 servings.

NUTRITIONAL COMPARISON (per serving):
"Traditional" Dutch Pancake = 364 calories, 34 carbs, 1 fiber
"Healthified" Dutch Pancake = 155 calories, 7 carbs, 3.25 fiber (using Almond milk)

FRENCH TOAST WITHOUT THE BREAD!

1 eggplant
Iodized Sea salt
2 eggs
1 tsp vanilla
Stevia Glycerite to taste
butter
cinnamon (optional)

Peel eggplant and cut into slices. Sprinkle a small amount of salt on the eggplant. Turn eggplant pieces over and sprinkle a small amount on the other side. Let eggplant rest for two minutes. Mix eggs, vanilla, cinnamon and stevia in a bowl. Melt butter in frying pan on med. heat.
Put your eggplant in egg mixture and poke holes into it with a knife or fork. This allows the mixture to permeate the eggplant. Cook "French toast" until golden brown. Then flip and do the same on the other side. Top with cinnamon, nutmeg, cream cheese, nut butter or low sugar fruit. Makes 2 servings.

NUTRITIONAL COMPARISON (per serving):
Using White Bread = 170 calories, 23 carbs, 3 fiber
Using EGGPLANT = 90 calories, 6 carbs, 3 fiber

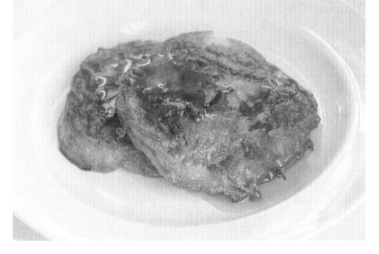

SCRUMPTIOUS SCONES

2 cups blanched almond flour
1/4 cup Erythritol and 1 tsp Stevia Glycerite
1 tsp baking powder
1/4 tsp baking soda
1/2 tsp Celtic sea salt
8 TBS unsalted butter, frozen
1/2 cup unsweetened vanilla almond milk
1 egg

Adjust oven rack to lower-middle position and preheat oven to 400 degrees F. In a medium bowl, mix almond flour, sweetener, baking powder, baking soda and salt. CUT butter with a knife into 1/2 cm squares; use your fingers to work in butter (mixture should resemble coarse meal). In a small bowl, whisk almond milk and egg until smooth. Using a fork, stir egg mixture into almond flour mixture until large dough clumps form. Use your hands to press the dough against the bowl into 8 balls. Place on a cookie sheet (preferably lined with parchment paper), about 2 inches apart. Bake until golden, about 13 to 15 minutes. Cool for 5 minutes and serve warm or at room temperature. Makes 8 servings.

NUTRITIONAL COMPARISON (per scone):
Traditional Scone = 319 calories, 41.1 carbs, 1.2 fiber
"Healthified" Scones = 271 calories, 6.25 carbs, 3g fiber

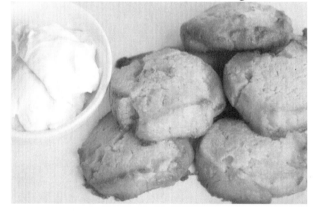

BREAKFAST HOT POCKET

3 eggs, separated
1/2 cup unflavored whey protein
3 oz. cream cheese, room temperature
1/2 tsp onion powder (optional)
Filling:
6 eggs, scrambled
6 slices bacon, cooked (or ham)
6 (1 oz.) slices cheddar cheese

Separate the eggs (save the yolks for a different recipe...crème brule???), and whip the whites for a few minutes until VERY stiff. Slowly fold in the whey protein and onion powder if using. Then slowly fold in the cream cheese into the whites (making sure the whites don't fall). Grease a cookie sheet very well. Spoon the mixture onto the pan making 6 large molds. Place a scrambled egg, cheese and chopped ham or bacon on each mold. Top with additional egg white batter and smooth the top with a spatula. Bake at 375 degrees F for 25 minutes until lightly browned. Enjoy! Makes 6 LARGE servings.

NUTRITIONAL COMPARISON (per pocket)
Store Bought Hot Pocket = 310 calories, 36 carbs, 3 fiber
"Healthified" Hot Pocket = 283 calories, 1 carb, trace fiber

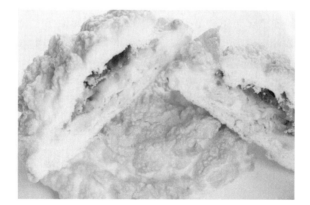

6 large egg yolks
1/4 cup lemon juice
2 TBS Dijon mustard
1 1/2 cups melted butter
1/2 tsp salt
1/8 tsp fresh ground pepper
1/8 tsp cayenne
3 cups Crab, or ham slices
12 large eggs
1 large eggplant (cut into
"English muffin" shapes)

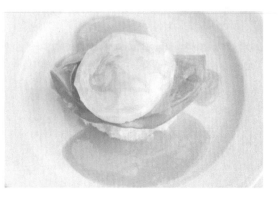

Make hollandaise sauce: In the bottom of a double boiler or in a medium saucepan, bring 1 in. of water to a simmer over high heat and adjust heat to maintain simmer. Put egg yolks, lemon juice, and mustard in top of a double boiler or in a round-bottomed medium bowl and set over simmering water. Whisk yolk mixture to blend. Whisking constantly, add butter in a slow, steady stream (about 90 seconds). Cook sauce, whisking, until it reaches 140°, then adjust heat to maintain temperature. Add salt, pepper, and cayenne and continue whisking until thick, about 3 minutes. Adjust seasonings to taste. Remove from stove and set aside. Preheat oven to 450 degrees F. Cut eggplant into "English muffins" (I used a round cookie cutter) and arrange on a baking sheet in a single layer. Sprinkle with salt and bake until toasted, about 5 minutes. Put 2 muffin halves on each plate and top with crab (or a slice of ham), dividing evenly. Poach eggs: Bring 1 in. water to boil in a 12-in.-wide pan. Lower heat so that small bubbles form on the bottom of the pan and break to the surface only occasionally. Crack eggs into water 1 at a time, holding shells close to the water's surface and letting eggs slide out gently. Poach eggs, in 2 batches to keep them from crowding, 3 to 4 minutes for soft-cooked. Lift eggs out with a slotted spoon, pat dry and place 1 egg on each crab-topped eggplant. Top with hollandaise. Serves 6.

Nutritional Information (with 4 TBS of hollandaise) = 424 Calories, 5g Carbs, 3g fiber

EGGS IN A FRAME

1 wide eggplant, cut into round or square bread-like shapes
4 eggs
Coconut oil or ghee
Celtic sea salt and pepper

Peel and cut eggplant into bread-like shapes. Then cut a hole in the middle of the eggplant for the egg. Heat a pan with oil, once hot add the eggplant to fry. Fry on both sides for 2 minutes or until soft. Crack egg into the empty hole in the eggplant and fry until the egg is done to your liking and enjoy! Serves 4.

NUTRITIONAL COMPARISON (per serving):
Using White Bread = 170 calories, 23 carbs, 3 fiber
Using EGGPLANT = 90 calories, 6 carbs, 3 fiber

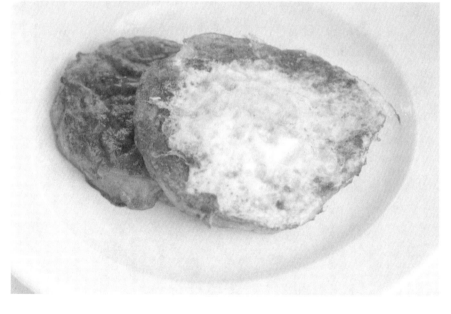

CREAM OF "WHEAT" CEREAL

3/4 cup of warm unsweetened vanilla or chocolate almond milk
2 to 4 TBS freshly ground flaxseeds (or more for a thicker "cereal")
1 scoop vanilla or chocolate whey protein (Jay Robb)
1 TBS vanilla extract
1 drop of Stevia Glycerite
1/2 tsp of nutmeg
1/2 tsp cinnamon
Optional: coconut flakes, nuts or peanut butter
Thicker Option: add 1/4 tsp of guar gum or xanthan gum (thickeners)

Combine warm milk, flax, whey, vanilla, stevia, cinnamon and nutmeg (and other toppings) in a bowl. Stir well and let sit for a few minutes until the "oatmeal" thickens. Enjoy! Serves 1.

NUTRITIONAL COMPARISON (per serving):
Traditional Cream of Wheat with Skim Milk = 230 calories, 39.6 carbs, 1.3 fiber, 12 protein
"Healthified" Cream of Wheat = 230 calories, 5g carbs, 4g fiber, 29g protein

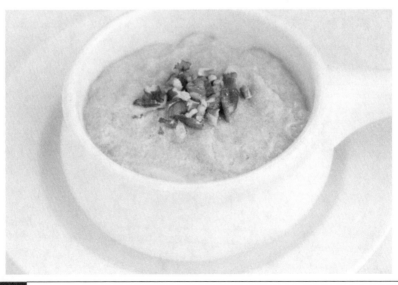

1/2 cup Jay Robb vanilla whey
3/4 cup blanched almond flour
1/4 tsp baking soda
1/4 tsp Celtic sea salt
1/4 cup butter
4 drops of Stevia Glycerite
2 TBS vanilla almond milk OR water(just
enough to hold dough together)
1 large egg (to brush on pastry)
Filling:
Nature's Hollow Jelly
Alternate fillings: 9 TBS of ChocoPerfection bar, 9 TBS
Homemade Nutella (pg. 224)

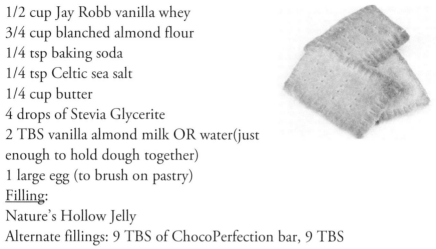

Preheat the oven to 350 degrees F. In a medium bowl, stir together the whey, almond flour, baking soda and salt. Cut in the butter until the butter lumps are smaller than peas. Stir in the almond milk (or water) and sweetener to form a stiff dough. On parchment paper, place 10 balls of dough a few inches apart. Shape with hands into rectangle shapes (size of a Pop Tart). Beat the egg and brush it over the entire surface of the rectangles. Even the "insides" of the tart; the egg is to help glue the lid on. Place a heaping tablespoon of filling into the center of each rectangle, keeping a bare 1/2-inch perimeter around it. Place a second rectangle of dough atop the first, using your fingertips to press firmly around the pocket of filling, sealing the dough well on all sides. Press the tines of a fork all around the edge of the rectangle. Repeat with remaining tarts. Gently place the tarts on a lightly greased or parchment-lined baking sheet. Prick the top of each tart multiple times with a fork; you want to make sure steam can escape, or the tarts will become fluffy pillows instead of flat toaster pastries (my mistake number 1). Bake for 10-12 minutes in the preheated oven, until edges are lightly browned. Cool in oven to crisp up. Serves 5.

NUTRITIONAL COMPARISON (per serving):
Kellogg's Pop Tart = 210 calories, 37 carbs, 1 fiber, 2 protein
Healthified Pop Tart = 199 calories, 3.8 carbs, 1.8 fiber

Strudel:

4 eggs

4 TBS coconut flour

1 tsp Stevia Glycerite

1 tsp aluminum free baking powder

2 TBS butter or coconut oil

1 tsp vanilla

Filling:

Walden Farms Jelly (I used raspberry)

Topping:

4 TBS Cream cheese

1/2 tsp Stevia Glycerite (if desired)

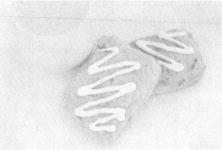

Preheat oven to 300 degrees F. Combine all the strudel ingredients and combine until smooth. Using tinfoil, form 4 rectangular shaped cups to place the dough, folding up the sides. Bake for 10 minutes or until a toothpick comes out clean. Cool, then using a knife, place a slit in the end and open the middle (without cutting the sides or other end). Place the Walden Farms Jelly in a ziplock. Squish around until it is a mush. Squeeze into the corner of the bag. Cut a tiny hole in the corner and squeeze into the strudel. Place the cream cheese in a ziplock. Squish around until it is a mush. Squeeze into the corner of the bag. Cut a tiny hole in the corner and squeeze onto the top just like you would with a "toaster strudel" frosting.

NUTRITIONAL COMPARISON:

Pillsbury Toaster Strudel = 190 Calories, 25 carbs, 1 fiber, 2 protein

"Healthified" Toaster Strudel = 185 calories, 5.5 carbs, 3 fiber, 8 protein

HEALTHY HASHBROWNS

1 cup shredded turnips OR Daikon radish
2 TBS coconut oil (I used ghee...clarified butter)
Sea salt and pepper to taste

Shred turnips or Daikon (let sit overnight in a bowl of chicken broth if possible). Heat oil in a skillet over medium-low heat. Add 1 cup vegetable to the pan and form a circle with the spatula. Fry for 6-10 minutes. When firm enough, flip the patty. Cook for 5 minutes, or until golden. If the patty falls apart, scramble the contents for loose hash browns, and stir occasionally until a golden color.

NUTRITIONAL COMPARISON (per cup):
Potato Hash browns = 116 calories, 28 carbs, 2 sugar, 4 fiber
Turnip Hash browns = 36 calories, 8 carbs, 5 sugar, 2 fiber
Daikon Hash brown = 30 calories, 2 carb, 1 fiber

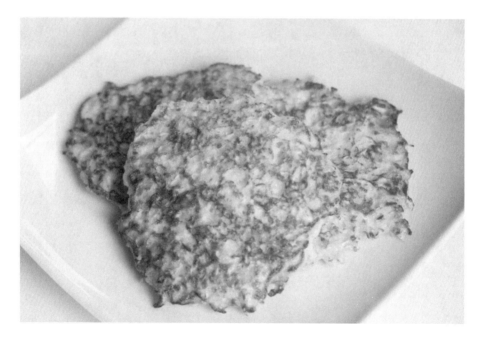

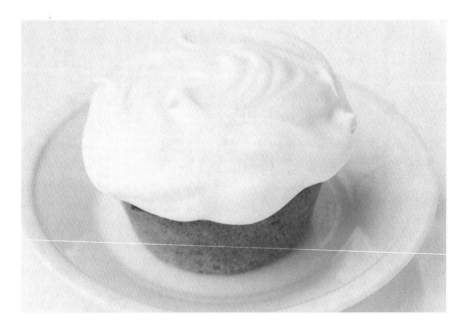

CINNAMON ROLLS

1/2 cup blanched Almond Flour
1/2 cup vanilla whey protein
1 tsp baking powder
3 TBS butter, softened
1 egg

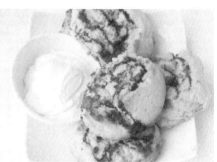

Preheat oven to 350 degrees F. Sift almond flour with whey and baking powder. Add the rest of the ingredients together until you have a smooth dough. Place a sheet of plastic wrap on counter, spray with cooking spray. Place dough on greased plastic, push the dough down a bit, and spray with another layer of olive oil. Top with another sheet of plastic wrap. Roll the dough out with a rolling pin until a long rectangle shape (9x12) or so. Then remove the top layer of plastic.

Cinnamon filling:
3 TBS Butter, softened
3 TBS Cinnamon
3 TBS Erythritol and 1/4 tsp Stevia Glycerite

Mix all ingredients together and spread evenly over the dough...make sure the top layer of plastic is off:) Roll up dough using the edge of the plastic to make a tight log. Cut into 2 inch pieces. Bake for 8 minutes or until baked through (insert a toothpick to check doneness...the toothpick should come out clean).

Top with cream cheese frosting:
6 TBS cream cheese, softened
3 TBS butter, softened
2 TBS Erythritol and 1/4 tsp Stevia Glycerite)
A little almond milk (to thin it out, if desired)

NUTRITIONAL COMPARISON: Make 6 Rolls
Cinnabon Cinnamon Roll = 730 calories, 119 carbs, trace fiber...YIKES!
"Healthified" Roll with frosting: 323 calories, 3 carbs, 1 fiber
"Healthified" Roll without frosting: 172 calories, 2 carbs, 1 fiber

CINNAMON BREAD

9 eggs, separated
1 1/2 cup vanilla whey protein or egg white protein
4-8TBS Cinnamon (depends on how much you like cinnamon!)

Preheat the oven to 375 degrees F. Separate the eggs and whip the whites until very stiff. Slowly add in the whey protein. Blend until smooth and then very gently add in the yolks (Yolks are optional) (try to keep the whites fluffy). Next swirl in the cinnamon. Grease a bread pan and pour the mixture into the pan. Bake at 375 degrees F for 45 minutes. Turn off the oven and leave the bread in to cool slowly. After an hour, take the bread out. Once totally cool, cut into 12 large slices. It makes great French toast.

NUTRITIONAL COMPARISON (per slice):
Pepperidge Farm Cinnamon Bread = 80 calories, 15 carbs, trace fiber
"Healthified" Bread = 47 calories, trace carbohydrates

GARLIC BREAD

3 eggs, separated
3 oz. cream cheese
1/4 cup parmesan cheese
1 tsp garlic powder

Separate the eggs, and whip the whites for a few minutes until VERY stiff. In a separate bowl, mix the cream cheese and yolks until smooth. Fold the parmesan and seasonings to the whipped whites. Then slowly fold in the yolk mixture into the whites (making sure the whites don't fall). Grease a bread pan very well. Spoon the mixture into the pan and smooth the top with a spatula. Bake at 375 degrees F for 45 minutes until lightly browned. Completely cool, then cut into 12 pieces. I also spread a little butter on each piece and sprinkled with additional garlic powder and parmesan cheese. I tossed it back into the oven on a broil for 3 minutes until butter was bubbly and lightly browned. Serves 12.

NUTRITIONAL COMPARISON (per slice):
Pepperidge Farm Garlic Bread = 170 Calories, 24 Carbs, 2 fiber
"Healthified" Garlic Bread = 64 Calories; 1 Carb; trace Fiber

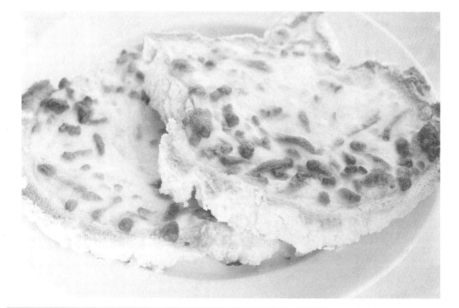

FRENCH TOAST BAGEL

3 TBS ground flaxseed
2 TBS coconut flour
1/2 t baking powder
4 egg, separated
2 TBS cinnamon
1/2 tsp Stevia Glycerite

Preheat the oven to 325 degrees F. In a medium-small bowl mix the dry ingredients - the golden flax meal, coconut flour, baking powder, cinnamon and stevia. Whip the egg whites until fluffy. Slowly add the yolks, and then the dry mixture. Allow the dough to sit for 5 minutes to firm up. Spoon the dough into a greased "donut" mold or shape into bagels on a cookie sheet. Bake for 30 minutes until the flax turns a darker golden shade. Allow to cool in the oven. Makes 6 bagels.

NUTRITIONAL COMPARISON:
1 Panera French toast bagel = 350 calories, **67 carbs**, 2 fiber
Small "LENDER's" Bagel = 140 calories, 29 carbs, 1 fiber
"Healthified" Flax bagel = 88 calories, 4 carbs, 2.7 fiber

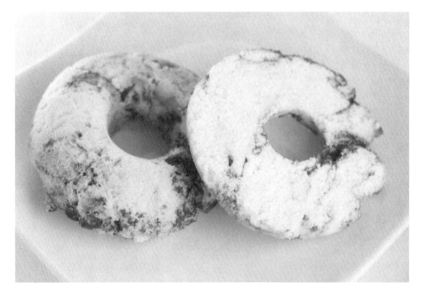

YORKSHIRE PUDDING

3/4 cup unflavored whey protein
1/2 tsp Celtic sea salt
3 eggs, separated
3/4 cup unflavored almond milk
1/2 cup pan drippings from roast prime rib of beef

Preheat the oven to 375 degrees F. Sift together the whey and salt in a bowl. In another bowl, beat the egg whites until very stiff. Set aside. In a separate bowl, mix together the yolks and almond milk until light and foamy.

Slowly stir the dry ingredients into the whites just until incorporated. Then add in the yolk mixture. Pour the drippings into a 9-inch pie pan, square baking dish OR I used large muffin tins (for individual servings). Put the pan in oven and get the drippings smoking hot. Carefully take the pan out of the oven and pour in the batter. Put the pan back in oven and cook until puffed and dry, about 20 minutes (or 10 minutes for muffin tin). Makes 8 servings.

NUTRITIONAL COMPARISON (per serving):
Traditional Pudding = 157 calories, 19 carbs, 0.6g fiber, 11g protein, 3.3g fat
"Healthified" Pudding = 45 calories, 0.9 carbs, trace fiber, 12g protein, 2g fat

OPTION: Fill "pockets" with pre-cooked breakfast sausage before baking.

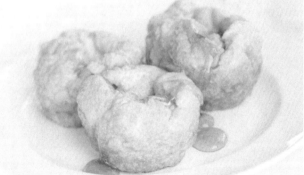

1/2 cup coconut flour
1/2 cup almond flour
1/8 tsp Celtic sea salt
1/2 tsp baking soda
1/2 tsp baking powder
1 1/2 tsp ginger
1 tsp cinnamon
5 eggs
1/2 cup coconut milk or
vanilla almond milk
1/4 cup coconut oil, melted
1 tsp Stevia Glycerite

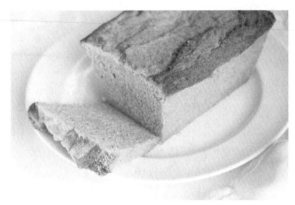

Preheat oven to 350 degrees F. Combine all dry ingredients in a bowl and whisk together. In a large bowl combine eggs, coconut milk, coconut oil and sweetener. Whisk together. Pour wet ingredients into dry ingredients, mixing thoroughly until smooth. Grease an 8×8 inch glass baking pan (or a small loaf pan) with coconut oil and fill pan with batter. Bake in a pre-heated oven for 40 minutes, or until firm to the touch, or when a toothpick or fork tine inserted in the center comes out clean. Cool and top with cream cheese frosting if desired. Makes 12 servings.

NUTRITIONAL COMPARISON:
Traditional Gingerbread = 208 calories, 29.8 carbs, 0.5 fiber
"Healthified" Gingerbread = 110 calories, 4.8 carbs, 2.5 fiber

ZUCCHINI MUFFINS

1 cup blanched almond flour
1/4 cup unsweetened cocoa powder
1/4 tsp Celtic sea salt
1/2 tsp baking soda
1/2 tsp cinnamon (optional)
2 eggs
1/3 cup Erythritol
1/2 tsp Stevia Glycerite
1 T Butter, melted
1 T vanilla almond milk
3/4 cup grated raw zucchini
1/2 cup chopped walnuts or pecans (optional)

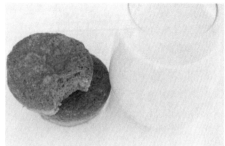

Preheat oven to 350 degrees F. Combine almond flour, salt, cocoa powder, cinnamon and baking soda into medium-sized bowl. Beat eggs and sweeteners for about 2-3 minutes. Then add butter and almond milk. Grate the zucchini. Squeeze out the water of zucchini if it seems wet, then measure out 3/4 cup of grated zucchini. Add 1/2 cup chopped walnuts or pecans. Stir the wet and dry ingredients together, only stirring enough to combine. Gently fold in the zucchini and nuts. Spray a 6 muffin tin with Olive oil spray, then divide mixture evenly into cups. Bake muffins about 45 minutes, or until top is browned and toothpick inserted into the center comes out clean. Yum! Makes 6 muffins.

NUTRITIONAL COMPARISON (per muffin):
Traditional Chocolate Zucchini Muffin = 217 calories, 29.7 carbs, 0.9 fiber
"Healthified" Zucchini Muffin = 157 calories, 6.7 carbs, 3.2 fiber

RHUBARB MUFFINS

1 cup flax seed meal

1/2 cup whey protein powder vanilla (Jay Robb)

4 TBS coconut oil or butter

1/4 cup Erythritol and 1/2 tsp of Stevia Glycerite

2 large eggs, lightly beaten

2 tsp baking powder

2 tsp vanilla extract

1/2 tsp salt

2 oz. chopped almonds (optional)

1/2 c unsweetened vanilla almond milk or coconut milk

1 cup chopped rhubarb

Pre-heat oven 350 degrees F. Mix all of the ingredients in a bowl, let stand for 3 minutes. Spray a 12 muffin pan with non-stick spray. Spoon batter evenly into muffin tins. Bake 25-30 minutes. Makes 6 muffins.

NUTRITIONAL COMPARISON (per muffin):
Traditional Rhubarb Muffin = 360 calories, 48 carbs, 4g fiber, 8g protein
"Healthified" Muffin = 236 Calories, 6 Carbs, 4g Fiber, 10g Protein

PUMPKIN MINI MUFFINS

1 1/2 cups blanched almond flour
1/4 tsp Celtic sea salt
1/2 tsp baking soda
1/2 tsp aluminum free
baking powder
1 tsp ground cinnamon
1/2 tsp ground nutmeg
1/4 tsp ground ginger
1/8 tsp ground cloves
2 TBS Butter or Coconut
Oil
1/2 cup Erythritol and 1/2 tsp Stevia Glycerite
3 large eggs
1 cup fresh OR canned pumpkin
Frosting:
4 oz. cream cheese
2 TBS unsweetened almond milk
2 drops Stevia Glycerite (to taste)

In a mixing bowl combine almond flour, baking soda, powder, salt, and spices. Mix butter, sweetener, eggs and pumpkin until smooth. Stir wet ingredients into dry. Grease or place paper liners in muffin tins. Spoon batter into the pan. Bake at 325 degrees F for 30-40 minutes. Cool and top with cream cheese frosting! To make frosting, mix together cream cheese, almond milk and sweetener until smooth; then dollop on top of muffins. Serves 6.

NUTRITIONAL COMPARISON (per serving):
Traditional Pumpkin Muffin = 403 calories, 73 carbs, 2 fiber
"Healthified" Muffins (4 mini muffins) = 198 calories, 7.7 carbs, 2.8 fiber

CINNAMON STREUSEL MUFFINS

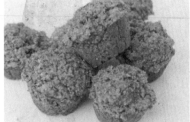

2 cup hazelnuts meal/flour
1 cup flax meal/ground flaxseed
2 tsp aluminum free baking powder
1/4 tsp Celtic sea salt
1 tsp cinnamon
1/2 cup Erythritol
1 tsp Stevia Glycerite
2 tsp vanilla extract
1/2 cup Unsweetened Vanilla Almond Milk
1/4 cup coconut oil or butter, melted
4 eggs
Streusel:
1 cup hazelnut meal (or other nut meal)
1/4 cup Erythritol and 1/2 tsp Stevia Glycerite
1 TBS cinnamon
1/8 tsp salt
1/4 cup chilled butter

Preheat oven to 350 degrees F. Grease muffin pan. In bowl, use pastry cutter to mix streusel ingredients until coarse and crumbly. You could do this in a food processor using pulse. Set aside. In another bowl, mix all muffin batter ingredients with whisk or spoon. Put a thin layer of batter (about 2 tablespoons) into each muffin cup. Add a tablespoon of streusel to each cup. Top with remaining batter. Then top this with the remaining streusel. Bake 20 minutes. Let cool slightly and remove from muffin pan to continue cooling. Serves 12.
NUTRITIONAL COMPARISON (per serving):
Traditional Boxed Cinnamon Muffin = 210 calories, 29 carbs, 0 fiber
"Healthified" Cinnamon Muffin = 182 calories, 2.5 carbs, 1g fiber

TORTILLA WRAPS

8 oz. cream cheese, softened
3 eggs
1 drop of Stevia Glycerite
1/2 cup ground flaxseeds
1/2 tsp aluminum free baking powder
1/2 tsp garlic powder
1/2 tsp onion powder
1/4 cup unsweetened almond milk

Pre-heat oven to 325 degrees F. Cut parchment paper into ten 12x12 inch squares and set aside. In a bowl, beat the cream cheese until smooth. Add the rest of the ingredients and blend until well mixed and resembles a pancake batter.

Place the parchment paper onto a plate to use as a guide for a round circle. Place 1/4 cup batter onto the parchment and spread the batter evenly and as thin as possible to make a 10 inch "tortilla". Place on a cookie sheet and bake for 10 minutes (or in microwave and cook on HIGH 1 minute). The tortillas should still look a bit doughy when they are finished. Let sit to cool. When cool enough to handle, peel the tortilla off the paper. Repeat with remaining batter. They should soften and become pliable after chilling several hours. They can be frozen. Makes 10 servings.

Nutritional Information (per serving) = 141 calories, 3g carbs, 1g fiber, 10g fat, 9g protein

TORTILLA CHIPS

1 Tortilla Wrap (previous recipe)
OPTIONS: add 1 tsp Mexican spices

Cut the tortilla wrap into about 6 wedges. Place on a microwave-safe dinner plate and microwave on HIGH about 1 minute, until golden brown and crisp. You may need to rearrange the chips for more even browning and add more time in 10-15 second increments or so at a time. Watch closely so they don't burn, although they do taste good when quite brown. Makes 1 serving

Nutritional Information = 141 calories, 3 carbs, 1g Fiber, 10g fat, 9g protein

CROUTONS

1 1/2 cups grated Parmesan cheese
1 1/2 cups almond flour
1/4 tsp Celtic sea salt
1/2 tsp garlic powder
3 TBS cold water to hold the dough together

Preheat oven to 350 degrees F. Pulse all the ingredients (except for the water) together in a food processor or blender. Add the cold water to the dough, a bit at a time, until the mixture is holding together well enough to work into a ball or two. Separate into two balls of dough, and place each ball on parchment paper, or other non-stick surface (which you will transfer to a baking sheet). Roll each dough ball out until flat and about 1/8 to 1/4 inch in thickness. Using a pizza cutter or knife, score the dough into squares, so you have squares that are the size of croutons. Bake for 25 minutes, or until croutons are browned. The darker, the crunchier. Cool and serve with a salad or soup.

Nutritional Information (per 8 half inch croutons) = 117 calories, 2 carbs, 1g fiber

HOMEMADE CROUTONS

Protein Buns
3 eggs, separated
1/2 tsp cream of tartar
3 oz. Sour Cream
1/2 cup Parmesan or whey
protein powder

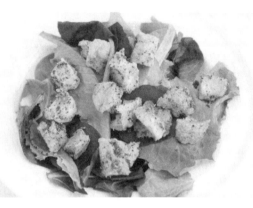

Preheat oven to 375
degrees F. Separate the
eggs and add sour cream to
the yolks. Use a mixer to combine. In a separate bowl, whip egg whites
and cream of tartar until stiff. Then add the Parmesan cheese. Using a
spatula, gradually fold the egg yolk mixture into the white mixture, being
careful not to break down the whites. Spray a cookie sheet with Olive oil
spray and spoon the mixture onto the sheet, making 6 mounds. Bake at
375 degrees F for 18 minutes, turn off oven. Keep oven shut, and leave
the buns in there for another 5 minutes or until cool. We use these for
our hamburger buns, but in this recipe we are going to make croutons
out of them.
Nutritional info (per bun): 80 calories, .9g carbs, 0 fiber, 6.3g protein

CROUTON RECIPE:
1 batch of protein buns, cut into crouton shapes
4 TBS butter
1-2 tsp garlic, minced

Preheat oven to 350 degrees F. Place the butter in a sauté pan on
medium heat until slightly brown, add the garlic and bread pieces to coat.
Place buttery croutons on baking sheet and bake for 15 minutes or until
crispy.

NUTRITIONAL COMPARISON (per 1 cup):
Pepperidge Farm Croutons = 186 calories, 25.4 carbs, 2 fiber, 4.3 protein
"Healthified" Croutons = 162 Calories, 0.9g carbs, 0g fiber, 6.3g protein

SUNFLOWER SEED CRACKERS

1 cup shelled sunflower seeds
1/2 cup grated Parmesan cheese
1/4 cup water
*Extra sunflower seeds (optional for topping)

Preheat the oven to 325 degrees F. Put the sunflower seeds and Parmesan in a food processor and process until the sunflower seeds are a fine meal. Add the water, and pulse until the dough is well blended, soft and sticky. Cover a cookie sheet with a piece of parchment paper. Roll the dough out onto the parchment, tear off another sheet of parchment, and put it on top of the dough. Use a rolling pin or your hands to press the dough into as thin and even a sheet as you can get. Take the time to get the dough quite thin--the thinner the better, so long as there are no holes in the dough. Peel off the top layer of parchment, then use a pizza cutter to score the dough into cracker shapes. Bake for 28-30 minutes, or until evenly browned. Peel off the parchment, break along the scored lines, and let the crackers cool. Store them in a container with a tight lid. *Option: Before baking press additional sunflower seeds into the batter for an extra crunch. Makes 6 dozen.

NUTRITIONAL INFO:
Each cracker = trace of carbohydrates, a trace of fiber, and 1 gram of protein.
The whole batch = 13 grams of digestible carbohydrates.

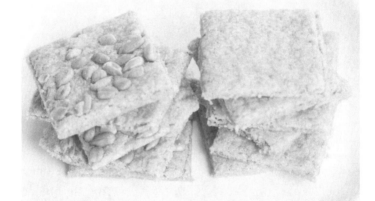

CHEDDAR CRACKERS

8 oz. sharp cheddar cheese, freshly shredded
3/4 cup almond flour
1/2 tsp Celtic sea salt
1/8 tsp favorite spice (cayenne)

Place the ingredients in a food processor and blend until the dough is well combined. Place the dough onto a large cutting board. Form a smooth ball of dough. Divide the ball in half. Roll each piece of dough into a ball and place back on sheet. Cover the balls with plastic wrap and take a baking powder can, that has about a 1/8" rim around the bottom, and press down firmly over each ball of dough. Be sure to press all the way down to the baking sheet. Peel off the plastic wrap and repeat until all the wafers have been shaped. Bake at 300 degrees F about 20-25 minutes or until lightly browned, checking frequently after 20 minutes. If there is any softness in the center, they are not done yet. Carefully remove them from baking sheet and cool completely on a rack. Can be frozen. Makes 48 crackers.

Nutritional Information (per 4 crackers) = 117 Calories, 2 carbs 1g fiber, 10g fat, 6g protein

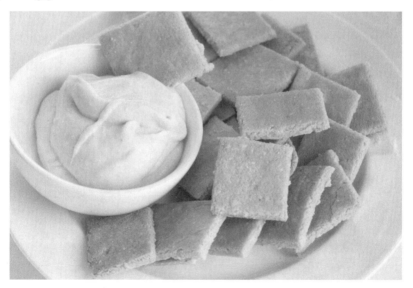

TOWNHOUSE CRACKERS

3/4 cup almond flour
1 drop Stevia Glycerite
1 egg white
2 TBS coconut oil or butter, softened
1/4 tsp Celtic sea salt

Mix all of the ingredients well in a small bowl. Put the dough on a well-greased sheet of heavy-duty aluminum foil, about 15x18". Cover the dough with a piece of wax paper that's been sprayed with non-stick spray. Very evenly roll out the dough to about 1/8" thick. Roll out in the shape of a square. Replace the wax paper and continue rolling until nice and even. Peel off the wax paper and use a pizza or ravioli cutter to score the dough into approximately 1-inch squares. Lift the foil and set it on the oven rack or on a baking sheet and bake them at 325 degrees F for 10-15 minutes, or until golden brown. Gently break them apart on the score lines and let cool. Can be frozen. Makes 48 crackers.

NUTRITIONAL COMPARISON (per 6 crackers):
Traditional TOWNHOUSE Cracker = 96 calories, 10.8 carbs, 1.2 fiber
"Healthified" Crackers = 90 calories, 2 carbs, 1g fiber, 8g fat, 3g protein

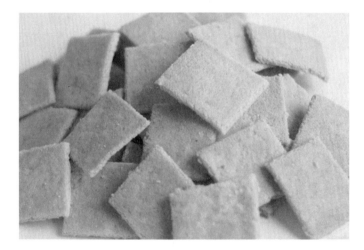

ALMOND CRACKERS

3/4 cup almond flour
1 drop Stevia Glycerite
1 egg white
3/8 tsp salt
1/8 tsp garlic powder
1/8 tsp onion powder

Place all ingredients in a small bowl and mix until well combined. Place the dough on a well-greased sheet of parchment paper, about 15x18". Cover the dough with a piece of wax paper that's been greased. Roll out the dough to about 1/8" thickness. Get the dough as even as possible so it bakes evenly. Peel off the wax paper and use a pizza or ravioli cutter to score the dough into 1-inch squares. Lift the parchment paper and set it on the oven rack. Bake at 325 degrees F for 10-15 minutes, or until golden brown. Check after 10 minutes, if the crackers at outer edge are getting brown, remove and continue baking the rest until golden. Break them apart on the score lines and let cool. They will keep for weeks in an airtight container. Can be frozen. Makes 48 crackers.

Nutritional Information (per 8 crackers) = 96 Calories, 3 carbs, 2g fiber, 7g fat, 4g protein

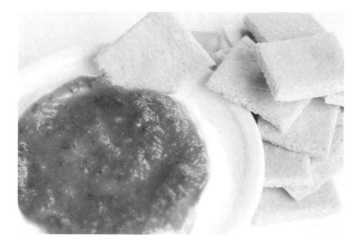

MINI PRETZELS

3/4 cup almond flour
1/2 cup unflavored whey protein
1/4 tsp baking soda
1/4 cup butter
1-2 TBS water (just enough to hold the dough together)
1/2 tsp salt
OPTIONAL: 1 egg, set aside

Preheat the oven to 325 degrees F. In a medium bowl, stir together the whey, almond flour, baking soda and salt. Cut in the butter using a pastry blender or your fingers until the butter lumps are smaller than peas. Stir in the water to form a stiff dough. Place the dough in a ziplock. Cut a small hole in the corner of the bag. Squirt the dough onto a cookie sheet, making shapes like a pretzel. (OPTIONAL: Whip egg in a small bowl, brush the egg wash on the pretzels and sprinkle additional salt on top.) Place pretzels 1 inch apart. Bake for 7-9 minutes in the preheated oven, until edges are lightly browned. Remove from oven to cool. Meanwhile, prepare a healthy dip like the Greek Avocado Dip (pg. 38) and Enjoy! Makes 12 servings.

NUTRITIONAL COMPARISON (per serving):
Traditional pretzels = 107 calories, 23 carbs, trace fiber
"Healthified" pretzels = 92 calories, 2.5 carbs, trace fiber

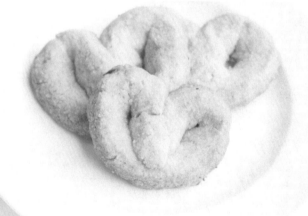

PINWHEEL BLUE CHEESE CRACKERS

1/4 cup butter, softened
8 oz. crumbled blue cheese
1 1/2 cup blanched almond flour
1/2 cup finely chopped walnuts
Pinch Celtic sea salt
Egg (for egg wash)

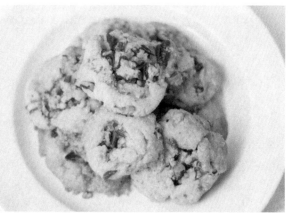

In a large mixing bowl, use a mixer to beat butter and cheese until smooth. Add almond flour and salt and mix until well-combined. Dump the dough onto a piece of parchment or a greased piece of plastic wrap, press it into a ball, and roll into a 12-inch long log. Brush the log completely with the egg wash. Spread the walnuts in a square on a cutting board and roll the log back and forth in the walnuts, pressing lightly, and distributing them evenly on the outside of the log. Wrap in plastic and refrigerate for at least 30 minutes or for up to 4 days. Meanwhile, preheat the oven to 350 degrees F. Cut the log 3/8ths-inch thick with a small, sharp knife and place the crackers on a sheet pan lined with parchment paper. Bake for 22 minutes until very lightly browned. Rotate the pan once during baking. Cool and serve at room temperature. Makes 36 crackers.

NUTRITIONAL COMPARISON:
Traditional Nut Thins = 130 Calories, 23 carb, 1g fiber, 3g protein
"Healthified" Nut Crackers = 70 calories, 1.1 carb, trace fiber

"RYE" BREAD

2 cups ground flax seeds
1 TBS baking powder
1 tsp Celtic sea salt
Added mixed dried herbs
6 eggs (separated)
1/2 cup water
1/3 cup coconut oil (or butter)
1 tsp Stevia Glycerite (optional, but creates a nice taste)

Place the egg whites in a mixing bowl and whip until stiff peaks form. Add the yolks, oil and water. Place the flax in another bowl and add baking powder, salt and herbs and mix.... Add the wet mix to the dry mix and mix thoroughly. Place the mix into a non-stick bread tin and bake 375 degrees F for 55 minutes. All ovens are different, so you will have to experiment a bit. Let completely cool before cutting.

Nutritional Information (per slice) = 102 calories, 4 carbs, 3.5 fiber, 5g protein

Ruben Toppings:
Nitrate free Corned Beef
Sauerkraut
Swiss Cheese
Homemade Mayo

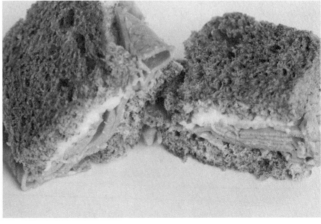

ZUCCHINI COCONUT BREAD

6 eggs, separated
3/4 cup loosely packed shredded zucchini
1/2 cup coconut milk (or 2 more eggs)
1/2 cup coconut oil (or butter) melted (plus extra for greasing pan)
1/4 cup Erythritol and 1 tsp Stevia Glycerite (or less to taste)
1 tsp pure vanilla
1 1/2 tsp cinnamon
1/2 tsp Celtic sea salt
3/4 cup coconut flour
1 tsp aluminum free baking powder
1/2 cup chopped pecans or walnuts (optional)
Unsweetened coconut flakes (optional topping)

Preheat oven to 350 degrees F. Grease a 9x5x3 inch loaf pan with coconut oil or butter. Separate 4 eggs into two bowls. Whip the egg whites until very fluffy. In the other bowl, blend together the 4 egg yolks, zucchini, oil, 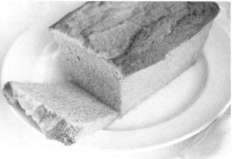 coconut milk, sweetener, vanilla, cinnamon, and salt. Then add the other 2 eggs (or 4 if not using coconut milk), one at a time, beating well after each addition. Combine coconut flour and baking powder and sift into batter. Blend until there are no lumps. Fold in nuts. Gently fold in the egg whites to the batter. Pour into a greased pan. Top with unsweetened coconut flakes and bake for 60 minutes or until an inserted toothpick comes out clean. Cool and enjoy! Makes 14 slices.

NUTRITIONAL COMPARISON (per serving)
Traditional Zucchini Bread = 377 calories, 43 carbs. 2 fiber
"Healthified" Zucchini Bread = 135 calories, 5.2 carbs, 2.3g fiber

TURTLE BREAD AND SPINACH DIP

<u>Dip</u>:

1 cup Spectrum organic mayonnaise

1 (16 oz.) container sour cream

1 (1.8 oz.) package dry leek soup mix

1 (4 oz.) can water chestnuts, drained and chopped

1/2 (10 oz.) package frozen spinach, thawed and drained

In a medium bowl, mix together mayonnaise, sour cream, dry spice mix, water chestnuts and chopped spinach. Chill in the refrigerator 6 hours, or overnight. Remove top and interior of turtle bread. Fill with mayonnaise mixture. Tear removed bread chunks into pieces for dipping.

<u>Turtle Bread</u>:

3 eggs, separated

1/2 tsp cream of tartar

3 oz. Sour Cream/cream cheese

1/2 cup grated Parmesan cheese, unflavored WHEY protein OR flaxseeds

Preheat oven to 375 degrees F. Separate the eggs and save the yolks for future recipe. In a bowl, whip egg whites and cream of tartar until VERY VERY stiff. Then add the Parmesan cheese. Using a spatula, gradually fold the sour cream into the white mixture, being careful not to break down the whites. Spray a cookie sheet with Olive oil spray and spoon the mixture onto the sheet, make into a "turtle" shape (OR make into 6 buns). Bake at 375 degrees F for 30 minutes. Keep oven shut, and leave the buns in there for another 5 minutes or until cool.

NUTRITIONAL COMPARISON (per serving):

Traditional Rye Turtle Bread = 166 calories, 31 carbs, 2.8g fiber

"Healthified" Bread (1/6 recipe): 80 calories, 0.9g carbs, 0 fiber, 6.3g protein

BABY "CORN" BREAD

1 can (15 oz.) baby corn, drained and chopped fine
1 1/4 cup almond meal
1 tsp Stevia Glycerite
1 tsp Celtic sea salt
3 1/2 tsp baking powder
5 eggs
1 cup vanilla almond milk
1/3 cup coconut oil or butter

Preheat oven to 400 degrees F. Lightly grease a 9 inch round cake pan or a bread pan. Drain baby corn and chop into small pieces. In a large bowl, combine almond meal, corn, sweetener, salt and baking powder. Stir in eggs, milk and oil until well combined. Pour batter into prepared pan. Bake in preheated oven for 20 to 25 minutes, or until a toothpick inserted into the center of the loaf comes out clean. Serves 12.

NUTRITIONAL COMPARISON:
Traditional Cornbread = 188 calories, 28.2 carbs, 1 fiber
"Healthified" Cornbread = 121 calories, 2.75 carbs, 1.1 fiber

NUTRITIONAL COMPARISON (per cup):
Corn = 132 calories, 30 carbs, 4 fiber
Baby Corn = 36 calories, 4 carbs, 4 fiber

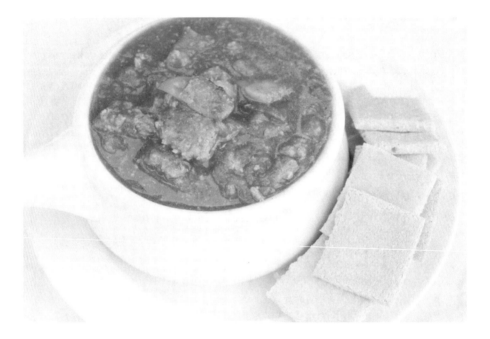

CAULIFLOWER SOUP WITH CAULIFLOWER BEIGNETS

Soup:
1/2 onion, finely chopped
1 garlic clove, finely chopped
1 strip of nitrate free bacon (cut into 1 inch strips)
13/4lb cauliflower florets, roughly chopped
13/4 pints chicken or beef stock
4 oz. cream cheese
Celtic sea salt and pepper (to taste)
Beignets:
3/4 cup cauliflower florets, roughly chopped
1/2 cup cold water
2 TBS unsalted butter, chopped
3 TBS freshly ground flaxseed
2 free-range eggs
2oz Gruyère cheese, grated
Celtic sea salt and pepper (to taste)
Coconut oil OR ghee or Expeller pressed Safflower Oil for frying

For the cauliflower soup, in a deep pot over medium heat, place the bacon, and add the onion and garlic and fry for 2-3 minutes, or until just softened. Add the chopped cauliflower and chicken stock. Bring the mixture to a boil, then reduce the heat and simmer for 8-12 minutes, or until the cauliflower is tender. Remove from the heat and set aside to cool. Carefully pour the soup mixture into a food processor and blend to a purée. Set aside, reserving the pan (you will return the soup to it). For the beignets, heat the oil in a cast iron "donut" hole-type pan (or a flat pan, but your beignets will be flat). Bring a pan of salted water to a boil, add the chopped cauliflower and cook for 2-3 minutes, or until just tender. Drain well, then refresh in cold water (if you use a microwave, you could steam it in that). In a separate pan, bring the water and butter to the boil and cook for 1-2 minutes. Remove the pan from the heat, then add all of the flaxseed meal and beat well until the mixture is smooth and well combined and thickens up a bit. Add the eggs, one at a time, beating each egg well until the mixture is well combined. Add the cooked cauliflower and the grated Gruyère and mix until well combined. Season to taste with salt and freshly ground black pepper. Carefully lower teaspoonfuls of the beignet mixture into the hot oil in batches. Fry for 2-3 minutes, or until crisp and golden-brown on both sides. Remove from the pan with a slotted spoon and set aside to drain on paper towel. Keep warm. Repeat the process with the remaining beignet mixture. When the beignets are ready, return the puréed soup mixture to the pan and add the cream. Season, to taste, with salt and freshly ground black pepper and bring to a boil for 1-2 minutes. To serve, divide the cauliflower soup equally among four serving bowls. Garnish the soup with the cauliflower beignets. Makes 4 servings

Nutritional Information (per serving of soup only) = 177 calories, 11 carbs, 3.7 fiber

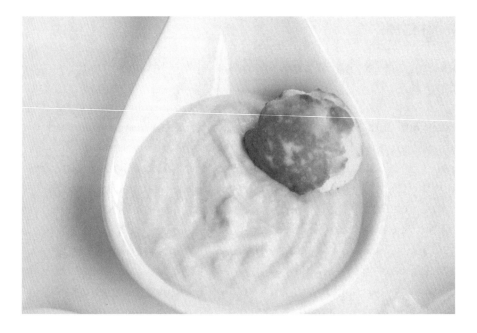

CLAM CHOWDER IN A "BREAD" BOWL

4 slices bacon, chopped into pieces
1/2 cup minced onion
1 cup diced celery
2 cups cubed Daikon
1 cup diced carrots
1/2 cup chicken broth
3 (6.5 oz.) cans minced clams
1/2 tsp fish sauce (optional Umami flavor)
1 tsp guar gum/xanthan (optional thickener)
2 cups heavy cream
2 cups unsweetened unflavored almond milk
2 TBS red wine vinegar
1 1/2 tsp Celtic sea salt
ground black pepper to taste

In a large skillet, fry the bacon, onion, celery, carrot and Daikon pieces in a pan until bacon is crisp. Drain juice from clams over the onions, celery, Daikon and carrots. Add chicken broth to cover, and cook over medium heat until veggies are tender. Meanwhile, in a large, heavy saucepan, whisk thickener into cream and almond milk, stir constantly until thick and smooth. Stir in vegetables and clam juice. Heat through, but do not boil. Stir in clams just before serving. If they cook too much they get tough. When clams are heated through, stir in vinegar, and season with salt and pepper.

Bread Bowl:
3 eggs, separated
1/2 tsp cream of tartar
3 oz. Sour Cream or cream cheese
1/2 cup Parmesan cheese, grated

Preheat oven to 375 degrees F. Separate the eggs and add sour cream to the yolks. Use a mixer to combine the ingredients together. In a separate bowl, whip egg whites and cream of tartar until stiff. Then add the

Parmesan cheese. Using a spatula, gradually fold the egg yolk mixture into the white mixture, being careful not to break down the whites. Form tinfoil into a "bowl" shapes (or use an oven-safe bowl-shaped pan). Spray tinfoil with Olive oil spray and spoon the mixture into the bowl, making 8 bowls. Bake at 375 degrees F for 18 minutes, turn off oven. Keep oven shut, and leave the buns in there for another 5 minutes or until cool. Nutritional info (per bowl): 80 calories, 0.9g carbs, 0 fiber, 6.3g protein

Nutritional Comparison: Serves 8
USING POTATOES = 501 calories, 28.4g carbs, 2.2 fiber, 23.9g protein
USING DAIKON = 450 calories, 8.4 carbs, 2.4 fiber, 23.9g protein

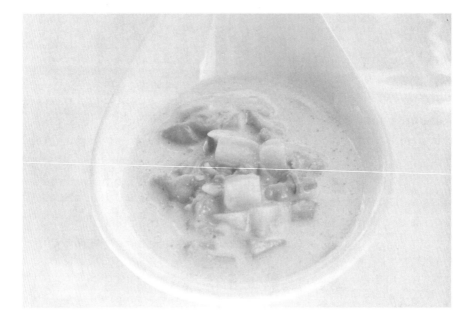

CHICKEN WILD "RICE" SOUP

I know the recipe sounds weird; instead of heavy cream, I used cream cheese. This added an amazing flavor without extra calories, 1 TBS of cream is 50 calories, 1 TBS of cream cheese is also 50 calories. Since you only need a small amount of cream cheese for the thickness and the flavor, you save a lot of calories this way.

1/2 cup butter
1/2 finely chopped onion
1/2 cup chopped celery
1/2 cup chopped carrots (optional)
1/2 pound fresh sliced mushrooms
6 cups chicken broth
2 cups chopped asparagus or Hearts of Palm(for rice)
1 pound boneless skinless chicken breasts, cooked and cubed
1/2 tsp Celtic sea salt
1/2 tsp curry powder
1/2 tsp mustard powder
1/2 tsp dried parsley
1/2 tsp ground black pepper
1 cup slivered almonds
1 cup cream cheese

In a large saucepan, melt butter over medium heat. Stir in the onion, celery and carrots and sauté for 5 minutes or until soft. Add the mushrooms and sauté for 2 more minutes. Slowly add in the chicken broth, stirring constantly. Bring to a boil, reduce heat to low and let simmer.

Next, add the Hearts of Palm (or asparagus), chicken, salt, curry powder, mustard powder, parsley, ground black pepper, almonds and cream cheese. Allow to heat through, and whisk to incorporate the cream cheese. Let simmer for 1 to 2 hours. Makes 8 servings.

NUTRITIONAL COMPARISON (per serving)
Traditional Soup: 529 calories, 28.7 carbs, 3.6 fiber
"Healthified" Soup = 365 calories, 6.25 carbs, 3.7 fiber

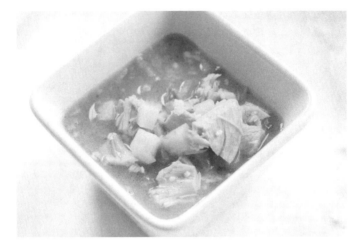

CRAB BISQUE

2 TBS Butter
1/8 cup chopped onion
1 clove garlic, minced
1 red pepper, chopped
1 cup asparagus, chopped
1 cup mushrooms, chopped
1 1/2 cup chicken broth
2 TBS Cream Cheese
2 TBS Brie Cheese (or more cream cheese)
1 can crab meat

Sauté onion, garlic, red pepper, asparagus, and mushrooms in the butter over medium heat. Let the vegetables "sweat" for 10 minutes. Slowly add the chicken broth, cream cheese and brie until melted. Then add the crab meat and serve. Makes 4 servings.

Nutritional Information (per serving) = 155 calories, 5.3 carbs, 1.95 fiber

BAKED "POTATO" SOUP

3 bacon strips, diced
1/2 cup onion, chopped
1 clove garlic, minced
1 tsp Celtic sea salt
1 tsp dried basil
1/2 tsp pepper
3 cups chicken broth
3 cups cauliflower flowerets
2 oz. cream cheese
1/2 tsp hot pepper sauce
Fresh Shredded Cheddar cheese
Minced fresh parsley

In a large saucepan, cook bacon until crisp. Drain, reserve 1 tablespoon drippings. Set bacon aside. Sauté onion and garlic in the drippings until tender. Stir in salt, basil and pepper; mix well. Gradually add broth and the cauliflower. Bring to boil; boil and stir for 5 minutes. Add the cream cheese and hot pepper sauce; heat through but do not boil. Remove from heat and place in a food processor to blend until smooth. Place in bowls, garnish with bacon, cheese and parsley. Makes 4 servings.

NUTRITIONAL COMPARISON (per serving):
Traditional Potato Soup = 323 calories, 21 carbs, 2.6g fiber
"Healthified" Mock Potato Soup =117 calories, 6.2 carbs, 2.77 fiber

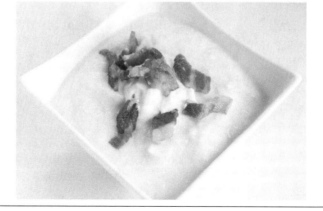

1/2 cup butter
2 TBS Coconut oil
4 cups sliced onions
4 (10.5 oz.) cans beef
broth
2 TBS dry sherry
(optional)
1 tsp dried thyme
Salt and pepper to taste
8 Protein Buns
4 slices provolone
cheese
2 slices Swiss cheese, diced
1/4 cup grated Parmesan cheese

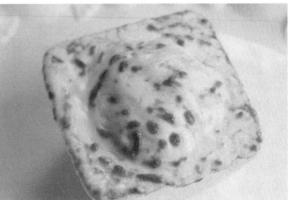

Melt butter with oil in an 8 quart stock pot on medium heat. Add onions and continually stir until tender and translucent. Do not brown the onions. Add beef broth, sherry and thyme. Season with salt and pepper, and simmer for 30 minutes. Heat the oven broiler. Ladle soup into oven safe serving bowls and place one Protein Bun on top of each. Layer each slice of "bread" with a 1/2 slice of provolone, 1/2 slice diced Swiss and 1 tablespoon Parmesan cheese. Place bowls on cookie sheet and broil in the preheated oven until cheese bubbles and browns slightly. Serves 8

NUTRITIONAL COMPARISON (per serving)
Traditional French Onion Soup (using wine and real bread) = 732 calories, 79 carbs, 4g fiber
"Healthified" French Onion Soup = 350 calories, 8 carbs, 1.7g fiber

CHICKEN "NOODLE" SOUP

4 cups zucchini or Daikon radish (cut into noodle shapes)
1 cup chopped celery
1/4 cup chopped onion
1/4 cup butter
4 cups chopped, cooked chicken meat
1/4 cup chopped carrots
12 cups chicken broth
1/2 tsp dried marjoram
3 slices fresh ginger root (optional)
1/2 tsp ground black pepper
1 bay leaf
1 TBS dried parsley

Peel and cut zucchini or daikon with the veggie swirler or by hand to resemble noodles. In a large stock pot, sauté celery and onion in butter until soft. Add chicken, carrots, chicken broth, marjoram, ginger, black pepper, bay leaf, and parsley. Simmer for 30 minutes. Add Daikon, and simmer for 10 more minutes. Serves 10.

NUTRITIONAL COMPARISON (per serving)
Traditional Chicken Noodle Soup: 227 calories, 19 carbs, 2 fiber
"Healthified" Chicken Noodle Soup = 120 calories, 4g carbs, 2g fiber

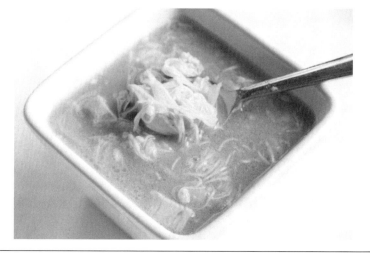

BROCCOLI CHEESE SOUP

1/2 cup butter
1 onion, chopped
1 (16 oz. package) chopped broccoli
4 (14.5 oz.) cans chicken broth
4 oz. cream cheese
1-2 cups sharp cheddar, shredded (depending on how "cheesy" you want it)
1 TBS garlic powder

In a stockpot, melt butter over medium heat. Cook onion in butter until softened. Stir in broccoli, and cover with chicken broth. Simmer until broccoli is tender, 10 to 15 minutes. Reduce heat, and stir in cheeses until melted. Mix in garlic powder. Enjoy! Makes 12 servings.

NUTRITIONAL COMPARISON:
Traditional soup with FAKE cheese = 491 calories, 34.9 carbs, 3 fiber
"Healthified" Broccoli soup = 321 calories, 6.5 carbs, 3 fiber

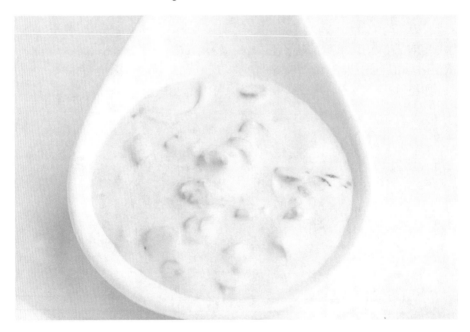

RATATOUILLE (FRESH FROM THE GARDEN SOUP)

1/4 cup coconut oil OR Ghee

1 lb. of yellow onions, chopped

3 cloves garlic, crushed

1 lb. zucchini, chopped

1 lb. yellow squash, chopped

Bell peppers, seeds removed, chopped into 1/2 inch square pieces:

--1 lb. green bell peppers

--1/2 lb. red bell peppers

--1/2 lb. yellow bell peppers

1 lb. eggplant, 1/2 inch cubes

1 lb. fresh ripe tomatoes

Celtic sea Salt to taste

2 sprigs thyme

1 bay leaf

1-inch sprig rosemary

3/4 cup vegetable stock (or quality tomato sauce with no added sugar)

Fresh ground pepper to taste

Preheat oven to 400 degrees F. Using a large oven-proof pan over medium high heat, sauté onions in 2 TBS oil until they begin to soften, about 5 minutes. Add garlic and reduce heat to low. While the onions and garlic are cooking over low heat, put 2 tablespoons of oil in another frying pan over high heat. As soon as oil is hot, add enough zucchini cubes all at once to cover the bottom of the pan. Keep on cooking over high heat, stirring until zucchini is lightly browned on all sides. Remove zucchini cubes and add them to pan with the onions. Repeat this process until all of the zucchini cubes have been cooked. Do the same with the yellow squash. Make sure to add a little oil between each new batch. Continue with the bell peppers, then the eggplant cubes, adding the browned vegetables to the onion pan as soon as they are cooked. When all the vegetables (except the tomatoes) are browned and in the pan with the onions, increase the heat to high and stir, making sure they don't stick to the bottom of the pan. Add salt to taste, thyme, bay leaf, and rosemary, the vegetable stock, and stir well. Place in oven, uncovered, for

30 minutes. (Alternatively you can cook them on the stovetop on low heat for 30 minutes). If using fresh tomatoes, boil water in a saucepan on stove. Remove stems from tomatoes, and crisscross the bottoms with a knife. Plunge into boiling water for a minute or two, until skin starts to fall away. Rinse in cold water and remove skin. Cut tomatoes in half lengthwise, remove seeds, chop coarsely, set aside. After the vegetables have been in the oven for a half hour, remove from oven, drain vegetables in a colander set over a bowl. Clean browned bits (if any) off bottom of pan with a paper towel. Return any liquid to the pan and reduce to a thick glaze over medium high heat. When all the juices have been reduced, return vegetables to the heavy pan. At this point the ratatouille should be moist and shiny, with very little liquid. Turn heat off. Add the chopped tomatoes and cover. If serving as a warm side dish, let the ratatouille stand for 10 minutes, just enough to "cook" the tomatoes. I like it best leftover when the flavors can "meld." When ready to serve, remove the bay leaf, and season to taste with salt and pepper. Serves 6-8.

Nutritional Information (per cup) = 151 calories, 11 carbs, 3 fiber, 12g fat, 1.9g protein

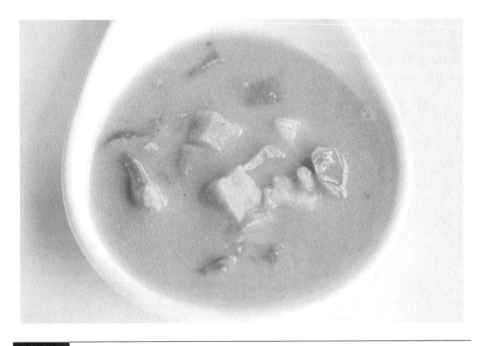

SPICY CHAYOTE SOUP

1 poblano pepper, roasted & skin removed

1 white onion, peeled and quartered

7 cloves garlic, peeled

3 medium chayote, trimmed, peeled and cut into eighths

1/4 - 1/2 pound fresh spinach, washed well and thick stems removed

4 cups chicken stock

3-1/2 cups unflavored almond milk

1 cup cream

1/2 tsp nutmeg

Celtic sea salt to taste (be generous, keep tasting)

OPTIONAL GARNISH

Sprinkles of cotija cheese

Sprinkles of nutmeg

In a large pot, combine the onion, garlic, chayote, spinach, chicken stock and poblano pepper flesh as it's prepped and bring to a boil. Cover, reduce heat to maintain a simmer and let simmer for about 30 minutes until the chayote is soft and cooked through. Remove from the heat. In batches, filling the blender no more than half full each time, purée the cooked ingredients until completely smooth. Return to the stockpot, stir in the milk and cream. Stir in the nutmeg and salt. Chill for 1 - 2 hours. Garnish soup servings with crumbled cheese and a sprinkle of nutmeg.

Nutritional Information (per cup) and 1/2 TBS cheese = 107 Calories, 8g Carb, 1g Fiber, 6g Protein, 10g Fat

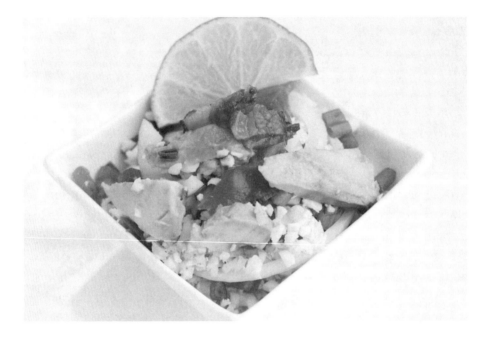

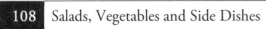

CAULIFLOWER GRATIN: 2 WAYS

2 large heads cauliflower, cut into 1-inch florets
4 TBS butter or coconut oil (divided)
1 TBS Celtic sea salt
2 tsp dry mustard
1 cup chicken broth
3 oz. cream cheese
2 cups freshly grated
fontina cheese (or other
soft white cheese)
2 cup freshly grated sharp
cheddar
Freshly ground black
pepper, to taste
3 TBS freshly grated
Parmesan cheese

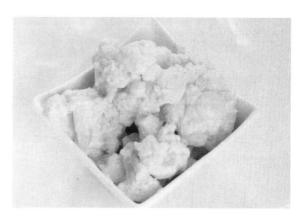

OPTION 1: Preheat oven to 400 degrees F and line a baking sheet with foil. In a large bowl, combine cauliflower, 2 TBS melted butter, salt and toss to combine. Place on baking sheet and roast until desired degree of tenderness (about 10 minutes for crisp tender, 20 for very tender). Remove from oven and place cauliflower in gratin pan.

OPTION 2: Bring a large pot of chicken broth to a boil. Place cauliflower in the broth and boil for 5 minutes or until tender. Remove from heat and strain the cauliflower well. Place in gratin pan. Meanwhile, in medium sauce pan over medium low heat, melt 2 TBS butter. Whisk constantly until starting to lightly brown, about 2 minutes, and slowly add chicken broth, dry mustard and cream cheese. Once completely combined, add shredded cheese and stir to combine until smooth.

Pour cheese mixture over top of cauliflower, sprinkle Parmesan cheese on top if using, and place in oven on middle rack. Turn broiler on low and cook until cheese sauce bubbles slightly. Remove from oven and serve immediately. Makes 8 servings).

NUTRITIONAL COMPARISON (per serving):
Using Potatoes: 499 calories, 49.3 carbs, 4.4 fiber
Using Cauliflower: 332 calories, 3.8 carbs, 1.7 fiber

DAIKON CHIPS

1 large daikon
1/4 cup coconut oil (or sesame oil)
Celtic sea salt (to taste)

Slice the daikon into 1/4 inch slices. In a large frying pan heated to medium and add half of the oil. Once the oil is hot, place the medallions in a single layer in the pan. Fry until they start to turn golden brown on the edges. Flip them, and cook until golden brown on the other side. Remove from heat, and arrange on a paper towel, sprinkle with a little salt, and enjoy!

NUTRITIONAL COMPARISON (per 1 cup):
Potato = 166 calories, 28 carbs, 4 fiber
Daikon = 30 calories, 2 carb, 1 fiber

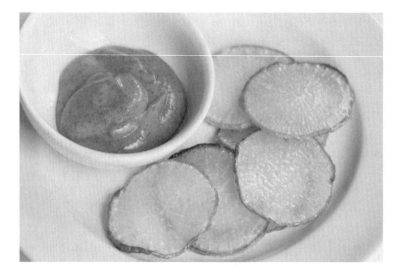

EGGPLANT CHIPS

1/4 cup Parmesan cheese, grated
1 tsp leaves Italian seasoning
1 tsp garlic powder
1 TBS coconut oil or butter (melted)
1 unpeeled eggplant, thinly sliced

Pre-heat oven to 375 degrees F. Pour melted oil on cookie sheet and sprinkle with the garlic powder. Swoosh the cookie sheet around to mix and coat the sheet well. Slice eggplant into about 1/4" or 1/8" thick rounds, depending on your taste and kitchen tools. Place eggplant slices on cookie sheet. Rub each slice into the oil and garlic powder coated cookie sheet, then turn each slice over and rub around to coat the other side. Sprinkle lightly with half of the Italian seasoning and Parmesan cheese. Turn over gently and sprinkle remaining Italian seasoning and Parmesan cheese on other side of rounds. Bake for about 10 to 15 minutes, depending on thickness, on each side. (Turn over when browned on the bottom). Note: this is a recipe you really need to watch cooking to see how well it is browning. They are done when they look caramelized on each side.

NUTRITIONAL COMPARISON (per cup):
Potato = 116 calories, 28 carbs, 4 fiber
Eggplant = 20 calories, 5 carbs, 3 fiber

"BREADSTICKS" WITH MARINARA

1 eggplant, peeled and cut into "breadstick" shapes
2 eggs beaten
1/2 cup Parmesan cheese, grated
1/2 cup almond flour
Italian spices
Marinara sauce (no sugar) for dipping
Expeller pressed Safflower Oil

In a bowl, whisk eggs. Set aside. In another bowl mix almond flour, cheese and spices. Place eggplant sticks into egg mix, then roll in almond flour mixture. Fry in a pan with safflower oil until golden brown (Safflower oil has a high smoke point so it won't become damaged).

NUTRITITIONAL COMPARISON:
Traditional Breadsticks = 150 calories, 20 carbs, 0 fiber
"Healthified" Breadstick = 59 calories, 1 carb, trace fiber

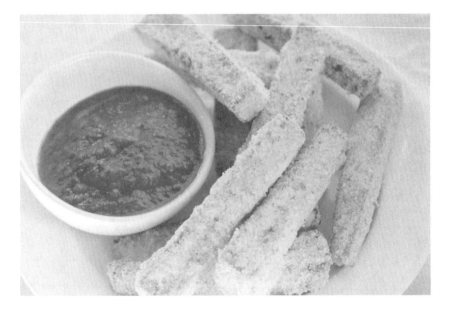

CHEESY BREADSTICKS

3 large eggs, separated
3 TBS sour cream
3 TBS Parmesan cheese
3 TBS unflavored egg white or whey protein
6 pieces of string cheese
Italian spices
No-sugar Marinara sauce for dipping!

Preheat oven to 350 degrees F. Separate eggs, whip whites until stiff peaks form. In a separate bowl add sour cream and Parmesan to the yolks (if using yolks). Slowly add the egg white or whey to the whites, followed by adding the yolk mixture. Shape the mixture around a piece of string cheese. Place on a greased baking sheet, sprinkle with Italian spices and bake for 13-15 minutes or until golden brown. Serve warm with marinara sauce! Makes 6 breadsticks.

NUTRITIONAL COMPARISON (per breadstick)
Traditional Stuffed Breadstick = 160 calories, 18 carbs, trace fiber
"Healthified" Stuffed Breadstick = 131 calories, trace carbs, trace fiber

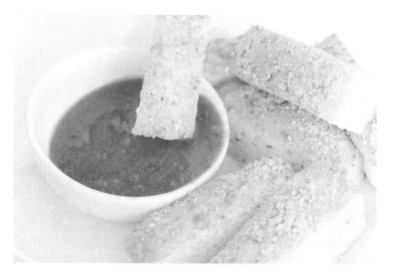

EGGPLANT FRENCH FRIES

2 Cups ground almonds (flaxseeds work here too)
Cayenne pepper to taste
Salt and pepper to taste
2 eggs, beaten
Healthy Cooking Spray
2 eggplants, peeled and sliced into fries

In a shallow bowl, stir together the almond flour, cayenne pepper, salt, and black pepper. Place the eggs in a separate bowl. Preheat oven to 400 degrees F. A few at a time, dip the eggplant pieces into the egg, then into the flour mixture, then back into the egg, and back into the flour mixture. Place the eggplant on a cookie sheet (I sprayed that with the cooking spray), then spray eggplant with a dusting of oil. Bake for 15 minutes or until crispy and brown.

Note: I reheated them in the oven the next day because the eggplant I used was HUGE, and they got even crispier and we like them better. Make sure to watch the ketchup...those sugars can really add up. Heinz makes a Reduced Sugar and it tastes great!

NUTRITIONAL COMPARISON (per cup):
Potato = 116 calories, 28 carbs, 4 fiber
Eggplant = 20 calories, 5 carbs, 3 fiber

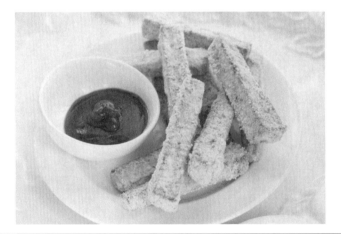

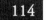

COCONUT ENCRUSTED CHICKEN SALAD

4 boneless, skinless chicken breasts
1/2 cup unsweetened coconut flakes
1/2 cup almond flour
Salt and pepper to taste
2 eggs
3 TBS coconut oil
8 cups of mixed salad greens
2 TBS olive oil
2 TBS lemon juice

Trim any remaining skin or white parts from the chicken breasts. Rinse under cool water and pat dry using a clean kitchen towel or parchment. On a chopping board, cut the chicken into strips somewhere between 1/2 an inch and an inch thick. Set aside. In a shallow dish, combine coconut flakes, almond flour and salt and pepper. In a bowl, crack eggs and beat lightly. Dip the chicken strips first in the egg and then roll in the coconut/almond flour mixture. Heat the coconut oil in the pan over medium-high heat and sauté the chicken strips until the exterior turns a golden brown and the inside is no longer pink. Remove from heat and place atop a bed of mixed greens. Drizzle with olive oil, lemon juice, and salt and pepper to taste and serve immediately. Serves 4.

Nutritional Information (per serving) = 600 calories, 7.9 g carbs, 3.8 fiber, 57g protein

GREEN BEAN SUSHI

1/2 pound green beans, trimmed
3 hard-boiled large eggs, quartered
2 TBS olive oil mayonnaise
1/2 tsp grated lemon zest
1/2 TBS fresh lemon juice
1/3 cup minced scallions
15 thin slices nitrate free ham or prosciutto (about 7 by 3 inches; 1/2 pound)

Cook green beans in a large pot of boiling salted water (3 tablespoons salt for 6 quarts water), uncovered, until just tender, 4 to 5 minutes. Drain, then transfer to an ice bath to stop cooking. Drain and pat dry. In a food processor, blend hard boiled eggs, mayonnaise, zest, lemon juice, scallions, 1/2 teaspoon pepper, and 1/4 teaspoon salt (or to taste). Place a sushi mat with slats running crosswise or a 9-inch square of parchment paper on a work surface. Arrange 3 slices prosciutto perpendicular to slats and slightly overlapping to form a 9- by 7-inch rectangle. Spread about 1 tablespoon egg mixture evenly across bottom half of prosciutto rectangle. Arrange beans on egg side by side and end to end, overlapping ends, in 8 tight rows parallel to slats. Spread another tablespoon egg mixture over beans. Roll up prosciutto and beans tightly with aid of mat. Transfer roll, seam side down, to a cutting board, then trim ends and cut crosswise into about 10 (3/4-inch) pieces. Make and cut 4 more rolls. Turn pieces upright to serve.

Nutritional Information (per 4 pieces) = 45 calories, 3 carbs, 2 fiber

SCALLOPED "POTATOES"

1 1/2 pounds Cauliflower stems,
thinly sliced
2 TBS butter, divided
1 cup chicken broth
2 cloves garlic, thinly sliced
Celtic sea salt and pepper to taste
2 cups shredded Cheddar cheese
4 slices provolone cheese
1/2 cup grated Parmesan or Romano cheese

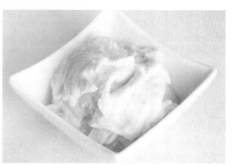

Preheat the oven to 325 degrees F. Grease a 1 1/2 quart or larger casserole dish with butter or nonstick spray. Layer half of the cauliflower slices in the bottom of the casserole dish. Dot with half of the butter cut or pinched into small pieces. Arrange half of the garlic slices over the slices, then pour half of the broth or heavy cream over. Sprinkle one cup of Cheddar cheese over the layer, and season with salt and pepper. Repeat layering of cauliflower, garlic, broth/cream and Cheddar cheese, then top with the slices of provolone cheese. Season again with salt and pepper. Bake for 1/2 hour in the preheated oven, then sprinkle the Parmesan or Romano cheese over the top. This will create a semi-hard cheese crust. Continue baking uncovered for another 30 minutes, or until cauliflower slices are tender when tested with a fork. Makes 6 servings.

NUTRITIONAL COMPARISON (per serving):
Using Potatoes and Heavy Cream: 686 calories, 24.3 Carbs, 1.8 fiber
Using Cauliflower and Broth: 210 calories, 1.7 carbs, trace fiber

CORN BREAD STUFFING

1 loaf of "baby corn" bread (see "Baked Goods" Chapter)
2 TBS butter
1/2 cup chopped celery
1 small onion
2 eggs, beaten
2 cups chicken stock
2 TBS poultry seasoning
Celtic sea salt and pepper to taste
OPTIONAL: peppers, mushrooms

Prepare the corn bread. Cool and crumble or cut into small cubes. Preheat oven to 350 degrees F. Grease one 9x13 inch baking dish. In a large skillet over medium heat, melt the butter and sauté the celery and onion until soft. In a large bowl, combine the celery, onions, 3 cups crumbled corn bread, eggs, chicken stock, seasoning, salt and pepper to taste; mix well. Place into prepared dish and bake at 350 degrees F for 30 minutes. Makes 6 servings.

NUTRITIONAL COMPARISON (per serving):
Traditional Corn Bread Stuffing = 364 calories, 52.8 carbs, 1.2 fiber
"Baby Corn Bread" Stuffing (6 servings)= 306 Calories, 6.8 carbs, 2.4 fiber
"Baby Corn" Bread Stuffing (8 servings) = 230 calories, 5.1 carbs, 1.8 fiber

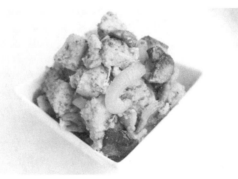

CHAYOTE SQUASH

1 TBS coconut oil or butter
2 medium chayote squash, quartered, seeded and diced
1 cup chicken broth
Celtic sea salt (to taste)
Fresh chives

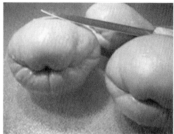

Heat a large skillet on medium-high and add the oil. When the oil is hot, add the chayote and stir to lightly coat with the oil. Cook through, stirring occasionally. Add the broth and simmer for about 5 minutes. Add the chives, let cook another minute. Remove chayote from broth. Enjoy! Makes 4 servings.

Nutritional Information (per serving) = 54 calories, 6 carbs, 3 fiber, 1 protein, 1g fat

"POTATO" CAKES WITH PEANUT SAUCE

1 1/2 pound Daikon radish or cauliflower
4 cups chicken broth or water
1 garlic clove, finely chopped
1/3 cup plus 1/2 cup finely chopped scallions, divided
6 TBS coconut oil or butter, divided
1/2 tsp ground cumin
1 medium tomato, chopped
3/4 cup unsweetened unflavored almond milk
1/2 cup NATURAL crunchy peanut butter
2 cups Munster cheese, coarsely grated (or other soft white cheese)

Peel daikon and cut into 1-inch pieces. Cover vegetable with chicken broth or cold water in a medium pot, then stir in 1 teaspoon salt and simmer until very tender, about 18 minutes. While the vegetable simmers, cook garlic and 1/3 cup scallions in 2 tablespoons oil in a small saucepan over medium heat, stirring, until softened, about 2 minutes. Stir in cumin and 1/4 teaspoon pepper and cook, stirring, 1 minute. Add tomato and cook, stirring, 2 minutes. Add almond milk and bring to a bare simmer, then remove from heat and stir in peanut butter until combined well. Keep peanut sauce warm, covered, off heat. Drain vegetable, then mash in a bowl (I used my Blend-Tec blender). Cook remaining 1/2 cup scallions with 1/4 teaspoon salt and 1/4 teaspoon pepper in 2 tablespoons oil in a small saucepan over medium heat, stirring, until scallions are softened, then stir into vegetable along with cheese. Form mixture into 8 balls and flatten each into a 3-inch patty. Heat 1 tablespoon oil in a 12-inch nonstick skillet over medium-high heat until hot, then fry cakes in 2 batches, turning over once, until crusty, about 6 minutes per batch. Add remaining tablespoon oil for second batch. Gently reheat peanut sauce, thinning to a creamy consistency with a little chicken broth or water if necessary. Season sauce with salt and serve with cakes.

NUTRITIONAL COMPARISON:
1 cup potato = 166 calories, 28 carbs, 4 fiber
1 cup Daikon = 30 calories, 2 carbs, 1 fiber
1 cup cauliflower = 28 calories, 3 carbs, 1 fiber

BROCCOLI CAULIFLOWER SALAD

10 slices nitrate free bacon
1/2 head fresh broccoli, cut into bite size pieces
1/2 head fresh cauliflower, cut into bite size pieces
1/4 Cup red onion, chopped
3 TBS white vinegar
1 drop Stevia Glycerite
1 Cup homemade mayonnaise
1 Cup sunflower seeds
2 hardboiled eggs, chopped (optional)

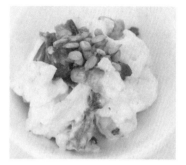

Place bacon in a large, deep skillet. Cook over medium high heat until evenly brown. Drain, crumble and set aside. In a medium bowl, combine the broccoli, cauliflower and onion. In a small bowl, whisk together the vinegar, stevia and mayonnaise. Pour over broccoli mixture, and toss until well mixed. Refrigerate for at least two hours. Before serving, toss salad with crumbled bacon and sunflower seeds. Makes 8 servings.

Nutritional Information (per serving) = 358 calories, 9 carbs, 4 fiber

BUTTERED BABY CORN

1 can of Baby Corn
Butter
A pinch of Celtic sea salt
A pinch of your favorite herb or spice (optional)

Melt butter in a pan. Sauté baby corn till slightly brown. Add a pinch of salt. Sprinkle herb (optional). Remove and serve.

NUTRITIONAL COMPARISON:
Traditional Corn = 132 calories, 30g carbs, 4g fiber
"Baby Corn" = 36 calories, 4 carbs, 4 fiber

TUNA "NOODLE" SALAD

4 cups Hearts of Palm

1/4 cup chopped dill pickles

1 stalk celery, chopped

Optional: 4 hardboiled eggs, chopped

1 (12 oz.) can tuna

1/2 cup Olive oil mayonnaise

1 pinch Celtic sea salt

Cut up the Hearts of Palm into "noodle-like" shapes. In a large bowl, combine the Hearts of Palm pieces, pickles, celery, eggs (if using) and tuna. Prepare the dressing by whisking together the mayonnaise and salt. Add to tuna mixture, and refrigerate for 1 hour. Makes 4 servings.

NUTRITIONAL COMPARISON (per serving)
Traditional Tuna Noodle Salad = 336 calories, 49 carbs, 4 fiber
"Healthified" Tuna Noodle Salad = 219 calories, 3.6 carbs, 1 fiber

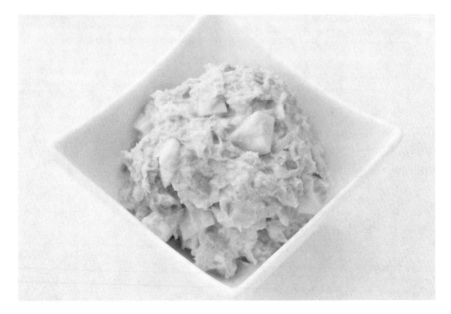

TURKEY-AND-SWISS CUPS

1 TBS olive oil mayonnaise
1 TBS cider vinegar
2 tsp Dijon mustard
1 1/2 oz. Gruyere cheese, cut into matchsticks
6 oz. peeled jicama, cut into matchsticks
1 small celery stalk, cut into matchsticks
8 radicchio leaves (from 1 small head)
6 oz. cooked sliced smoked turkey
Fresh chives, for garnish

Stir together first 3 ingredients (through mustard) in a medium bowl. Add cheese and next 2 ingredients (through celery), and toss to combine. Fill the radicchio leaves evenly with jicama and the turkey slices. Garnish with chives, if desired, and serve immediately. Makes 4 servings.

Nutritional Information (per serving) = 102 Calories, 8 carbs, 3 fiber, 11 protein, 2 fat

SEAFOOD SALAD

2 TBS olive oil
1 large onion, diced
1 pound large shrimp, peeled and deveined
1 pound scallops, rinsed and patted dry
1 (6 oz.) can crabmeat, drained and flaked
1 (12 oz.) can water packed tuna, drained and flaked
Celtic sea salt and pepper to taste
1 TBS seafood seasoning
1 cup olive oil mayonnaise, or to taste
2 TBS yellow mustard
1/2 tsp garlic powder, or to taste
1 tsp dried oregano
1/2 tsp ground turmeric
2 TBS white sugar
1 large green bell pepper, chopped
2 stalks celery, chopped
5 hard-cooked eggs, chopped
1 hard-cooked egg, sliced
1/2 tsp paprika, as garnish

Heat oil over medium heat in a large skillet and add onions, stirring until translucent, about 7 minutes. Add shrimp, scallops, crab meat and tuna. Cook until shrimp are pink and the scallops are opaque, 8 to 10 minutes. Season with salt, pepper, and seafood seasoning. Remove from heat. Whisk together the mayonnaise, mustard, garlic powder, oregano, turmeric and sugar in a large bowl. Mix in the bell pepper, celery and chopped eggs. Add seafood and toss until evenly combined. Garnish with eggs slices and sprinkle with paprika. Cover and refrigerate for 2 to 3 hours or overnight before serving to let flavors blend. Serves 30.

Nutritional Information (per serving) =132 Calories, 2.7 carbs, 0.3 fiber, 11.1g protein, 8.4g fat

COCONUT & CURRY BROCCOLI

1 TBS coconut oil
1 TBS garlic
12 oz. bok choy, stems chopped, leaves chopped separately
8 oz. broccoli florets
1 cup coconut milk
1/4 tsp Stevia Glycerite
1/4 tsp green Thai curry paste
1 TBS black sesame seeds

In a large skillet, heat the oil on medium heat. Once the oil is hot, add the garlic and cook for a minute. Add the chopped bok choy stems and cook for 5 minutes, while prepping the broccoli and leaves. Stir in the broccoli, stir to coat with oil. Let cook until broccoli is heated through. Move the vegetables aside, add the coconut milk, sweetener and curry paste, stir to mix. Stir together the bok choy stems, the broccoli and the bok choy leaves, coating with coconut milk. Reduce heat to medium-low, cover and let cook, stirring frequently, until broccoli and bok choy are both cooked clear through. Sprinkle with sesame seeds. Makes 6 servings.

Nutritional Information (per serving) = 120 Calories, 8g Carb, 3 g Fiber, 3 g Protein; 9 g Fat

SWEET "POTATO" CASSEROLE

3 cups mashed cauliflower

1 cup pumpkin (or more...if you want a deeper color)

1/4 cup Erythritol and 1/4 tsp Stevia Glycerite

-Or you could use Nature's Hollow xylitol pancake syrup

2 eggs, beaten

1/2 cup almond milk

1/2 tsp Celtic sea salt

1/3 cup butter, melted

1 tsp vanilla extract

Topping:

1/2 cup Erythritol and 1/4 tsp Stevia Glycerite

1/2 cup almond flour or almond meal

1/3 cup butter, melted

1 cup chopped pecans

Place cauliflower florets in a steamer basket over boiling water, cover and steam until very tender, 12 to 15 minutes. Place the cooked cauliflower in a food processor and blend until very smooth. In a mixing bowl, combine the cauliflower, pumpkin, sweetener, eggs, almond milk, salt, 1/3 cup butter and vanilla. Mix together and pour into a greased 13x9 inch baking dish. To prepare the topping, combine the sweetener, almond flour, 1/3 cup melted butter and pecans. Mix together and crumble over "sweet potato" mixture. Bake uncovered at 350 degrees F for 35 to 45 minutes. Serves 10

NUTRITIONAL COMPARISON (per serving):

Traditional Sweet Potato Casserole = 407 calories, 68.6 carbs, 2g fiber

"Healthified" Casserole = 190 calories, 5.3 carbs, 2.5 fiber

TURNIP GRATIN

2 TBS butter
2 1/2 pounds medium turnips, trimmed and left unpeeled
1 TBS chopped thyme
1/2 TBS chopped savory
1 1/2 tsp Celtic sea salt
1/8 tsp cayenne
1/2 cup heavy cream
1/2 cup beef broth
1 cup grated Parmigiano-Reggiano

Preheat oven to 450 degrees F with rack in middle. Melt butter in an ovenproof 12-inch heavy skillet, then cool. Slice turnips paper-thin with slicer, then arrange one third of slices, overlapping tightly, in skillet, keeping remaining slices covered with dampened paper towels. Sprinkle with about a third of thyme, savory, kosher salt, and cayenne. Make 2 more layers. Cook, covered, over medium heat until underside is browned, about 10 minutes. Add cream and broth. Continue to cook, covered, until center is tender, 20 to 25 minutes. Sprinkle evenly with cheese, then bake, uncovered, until golden and bubbling, 10 to 15 minutes. Let stand 5 minutes before serving.

NUTRITIONAL COMPARISON (per cup):
1 cup Potato = 116 calories, 28 carbs, 4 fiber
1 cup Turnip = 36 calories, 8 carbs, 2 fiber

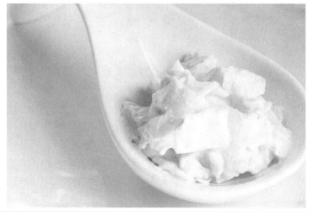

BRUSSEL SPROUT WITH PANCETTA

Water to steam
1 lb. Brussels sprouts
2 oz. thin-sliced pancetta
1 TBS garlic
8 fresh basil leaves, shredded
1 TBS coconut oil or butter
1 tsp balsamic vinegar
Salt to taste
Hot sauce to taste

Add water to a steamer and bring to a boil. Trim the sprouts: Slice off the base and remove the outer leaves. Cut each sprout in half lengthwise through the core, then make V-shaped cuts to remove the core. With your thumbs on the either side of the V, twist the sprout to open up the leaves a bit. Steam the sprouts for 5 minutes. Meanwhile, sauté the pancetta over MEDIUM fire in a small skillet until the edges have started to brown, breaking it into pieces with a spatula while it cooks. Add the garlic and cook for a minute. Drain the water from the steamer and return the sprouts to the hot pan. Stir in the pancetta and garlic mixture, including the fat in the skillet. Add the basil, oil (if using) and balsamic vinegar. Season with salt and hot sauce and toss well. Cover and let rest for 5 minutes. Toss again and serve. Serves 4.
Nutritional Information (per serving) = 111 Calories, 11 g Carbs, 4 g Fiber, 7 g Protein; 5 g Fat

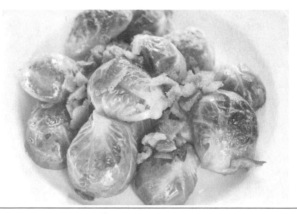

Salads, Vegetables and Side Dishes

SHREDDED BRUSSEL SPROUTS

4 cups water
1 TBS Celtic sea salt
1 pound Brussels sprouts
1 TBS coconut oil or butter (plus another 1 TBS later)
1 onion, chopped
2 cloves garlic, minced
Salt & pepper to taste
2 TBS balsamic vinegar
1/4 toasted walnuts (or toasted pine nuts)

Bring the water and salt to a boil in a large pot. Meanwhile, wash the sprouts and slice off a bit of the stem end. This will release the outer layer of leaves, go ahead and discard these. With a knife, cut an X into the core. (This helps heat get into the center core so they cook evenly.) Turn into the boiling water and cook until nearly done. (They'll finish in the skillet.) Drain. Slice cross-wise. In the same pot, heat the oil on medium heat. Once hot, add the onion and garlic, stir to coat with oil. Let cook until beginning to turn gold, stirring often. If needed, add another tablespoon of oil, then stir in the sliced Brussels sprouts. Let cook, stirring often, until sprouts begin to brown. Season to taste. Stir in vinegar and let cook a minute until liquid cooks off. Stir in walnuts and let warm through. Serve immediately. Serves 4.

Nutritional Information (per serving with walnuts) = 174 Calories, 15g carbs, 5g fiber, 6 g Protein, 12 g Fat

"POTATO" PUREE

1 head cauliflower, trimmed, cored, cut into florets
2 medium turnips, peeled and chopped
Salted water to cover
1 slice lemon
1 bay leaf
1/4 cup chicken broth (optional)
1 TBS fresh sage
Dash of Tabasco
Salt and pepper to taste
1 TBS butter

Bring the water to boil. Add the prepared cauliflower and turnips, then the lemon and bay leaf. Bring to a boil, cover, reduce heat to medium and cook until soft but not mushy. Drain and transfer to a food processor to puree. Add the herbs, Tabasco, seasoning and butter (slowly add the broth if it needs thinning). If the purée is too watery, return to the dry cooking pan and cook for a few minutes to cook off the excess liquid. Serve and enjoy! Serves 4 cups.

Nutritional Information (per cup) = 80 Calories, 10g carbs, 5g fiber, 4 g Protein, 3 g Fat

SPANISH "RICE"

1 head cauliflower, cut into florets
1 TBS coconut oil or butter
1 onion, chopped
1 green pepper, chopped
2 cloves garlic, chopped
8 oz. canned tomatoes, chopped
Salsa to taste
Salt and pepper to taste

Place cauliflower flowerets in a food processor and pulse until small pieces of rice.

In a large skillet, heat the oil on medium heat. Add the onion and green pepper and cook, stirring often, until golden. Add the garlic and cook for a minute. Add the tomatoes and stir in. Add in the cauliflower, stir it in and continue to cook. After cooking awhile, stir in the salsa. Keep cooking, keep tasting, adding more salsa and salt and pepper as needed. The dish is 'done' when the liquid has cooked off, the salsa and seasoning are perfect, and the rest of supper is done too! Makes 5 servings.

Nutritional Information (per serving) = 92 Calories, 15g carbs, 5g fiber, 4g Protein, 3g Fat

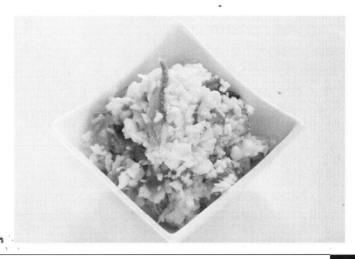

BACON CAROLINA "RICE"

1 (1/2-pound) nitrate free bacon, cut crosswise into 1/4-inch-thick pieces
1 1/4 cups finely chopped onion
2/3 cup finely chopped celery
2 garlic cloves, minced
1/2 tsp dry mustard
1/4 tsp cayenne
1/4 tsp hot smoked paprika
1/2 cup chicken broth
1/2 cup tomato sauce
3 cups "riced" cauliflower
2 TBS unsalted butter
1/2 tsp Celtic sea salt

Cook bacon in a 4-quart heavy pot over low heat until some of fat is rendered, about 5 minutes. Add onion, celery, and garlic and cook, stirring occasionally, until vegetables are softened but not browned, 7 to 8 minutes. Stir in spices. Add stock and tomato sauce and bring to a boil. Place cauliflower flowerets in a food processor and pulse until small pieces of rice. Stir in cauliflower rice and simmer, uncovered, stirring occasionally, until some of liquid is absorbed and cauliflower is cooked through, about 5-7 minutes. Stir in butter, salt, and pepper to taste, then remove from heat and let stand 5 minutes.

NUTRITIONAL COMPARISON (per cup):
White Rice = 242 calories, 53 carbs, 0 fiber
Brown Rice =218 calories, 46 carbs, 4 fiber
Cauliflower "Rice" = 28 calories, 3 carbs, 1 fiber

PESTO-RICE STUFFING

4 cups cooked cauliflower "rice"
1 cup pesto
1/2 cup pine nuts
8- to 10-pound turkey
Butter or coconut oil
Bacon slices

Place cauliflower flowerets in a food processor and pulse until small pieces of rice. Toss the cauliflower rice with the pesto and pine nuts and stuff the bird lightly. Close the vent and truss the bird. Rub well with butter or coconut oil. Place the turkey on its side on a rack in a roasting pan. Cover with slices of bacon and roast at 325 degrees F for 1 hour. Turn on other side and roast for another hour. Turn the bird on its back and roast with bacon covering the breast and legs until the bird is tender and done. Baste from time to time.

NUTRITIONAL COMPARISON (per cup):
White Rice = 242 calories, 53 carbs, 0 fiber
Brown Rice =218 calories, 46 carbs, 4 fiber
Cauliflower "Rice" = 28 calories, 3 carbs, 1 fiber

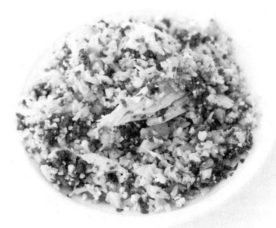

CREAMY PUMPKIN "RISOTTO"

4 cups finely chopped cauliflower, into "rice"
1/4 cup chicken broth
1 cup diced onion
1 cup thinly sliced mushrooms
1/2 cup canned pumpkin
1/2 cup unsweetened unflavored almond milk
1 tsp chopped garlic
1/4 tsp Celtic sea salt
1/8 tsp black pepper, or more to taste
2 wedges The Laughing Cow Creamy Swiss cheese
4 tsp Parmesan cheese
OPTIONAL: pumpkin seeds

In a food processor, pulse cauliflower into small pieces of "rice." In a nonstick pan, combine all ingredients except cheese wedges and Parmesan. Stir until well mixed. Bring to a soft boil. Once boiling, reduce heat to medium low and cover. Simmer for about 5 minutes, until veggies are tender. Add cheese wedges and Parmesan, and stir until evenly distributed. Season to taste with additional salt and pepper and top with pumpkin seeds if desired. Enjoy! Makes 4 servings (1 1/4 cup per serving).

NUTRITIONAL COMPARISON:
Traditional Pumpkin Risotto = 406 calories, 65.9 carbs, 2.9 fiber
"Healthified" Pumpkin Risotto = 222 calories, 4.15g carbs, 3.25g fiber

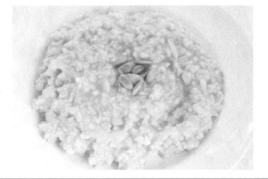

BAKED CHEESE "GRITS"

1 tsp Celtic sea salt
3 cups Cauliflower "grits"
1/2 stick (1/4 cup) unsalted butter
1/2 tsp black pepper
1 TBS chopped garlic
1 cup Cheddar, coarsely grated
2 large eggs

Preheat oven to 350 degrees F. Place cauliflower flowerets in a food processor and pulse until small pieces of rice ("grits").

Place "grits" in a saucepan, add butter, salt, pepper, garlic, and cheese, stirring until butter and cheese are melted. Lightly beat eggs in a small bowl, then stir into "grits" until combined. Pour into an ungreased 8-inch square baking dish (2 inches deep) and bake until set and lightly browned, about 1 hour. Serve immediately. I topped mine with Shrimp! Makes 4 servings.

Nutritional Information (per serving) = 284 Calories, 3.1 carbs, 0.9g fiber, 7g protein

NUTRITIONAL COMPARISON (per cup)
Traditional Corn Grits = 143 calories, 31.1 carbs, 0.1 fiber
Cauliflower Grits = 28 calories, 3 carbs, 1 fiber

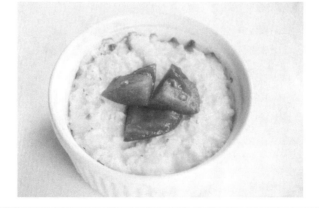

FRIED GREEN TOMATOES

1 large tomato (slightly green, yet soft)
1/2 cup almond meal (doesn't have to be blanched)
1 egg
1/2 tsp Celtic sea salt
Fresh ground pepper to taste
1/4 cup Coconut oil OR Ghee/Butter (for frying)
Optional: fresh basil from the garden

In a frying pan heat oil. Cut tomato into 1/4 inch slices. Break the egg and mix in a small bowl. Mix the almond meal (or other ground nut), salt and pepper (and other spices/herbs if desired) in another small bowl.

Place the cut tomato in the egg mixture, then in the almond mixture until well coated. Place in hot oil and fry until golden brown. Enjoy! Makes 4 servings.

Nutritional Information (per serving) = 204 calories, 4.7 carbs, 2g fiber

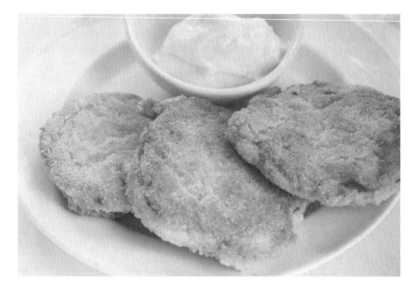

GREEN BEANS WITH BASIL

1 TBS coconut oil or butter
1 large onion
1 TBS minced garlic
1 pound green beans
1/2 cup chicken broth
1 tomato
1 cup fresh basil, chopped finely
Celtic sea salt & pepper

In a large, deep skillet with a cover, heat oil on medium-high heat. Chop the onion. Add onion and garlic to the skillet and cook until soft and just beginning to brown. While onion cooks, wash beans, break off stem ends and break each bean into about three pieces. Add beans and broth, tomatoes and basil to skillet, cover and bring to a boil. Reduce heat to medium and let simmer until beans are fully cooked, about 30 minutes, stirring occasionally. Season with salt and pepper and serve. Makes 4 servings.

Nutritional Information (per serving) = 95 Calories, 14g carbs, 5g fiber, 3g protein, 4g fat

CUCUMBER "BLT"

1 large cucumber
3 slices cooked nitrate free bacon, chopped into pieces
1/2 cup chopped lettuce
1/2 cup chopped baby spinach
1/4 cup diced tomato
1-1/2 TBS olive oil mayonnaise
Pinch Celtic sea salt
1/4 tsp freshly ground pepper

Trim the ends of the cucumber off, and slice in half lengthwise. Use a spoon to scoop out seeds and discard. Cook the bacon, chop, then combine with lettuce, spinach, tomato and mayonnaise. Season with salt and pepper. Divide BLT mixture between cucumber halves, mounding in hollowed areas. You can serve this as one large salad for yourself, or cut into smaller pieces for an appetizer.

Nutritional Information (per 4 inch slice) = 52 calories, 4 carbs, 1.9 fiber, 4 protein, 4g fat

CRUNCHY TOP "FAUX"TATOES

2 pounds "hash brown" turnips or cauliflower
1 whole onion, chopped
1 pound sharp cheddar cheese
1 16 oz. package sour cream
3 oz. cream cheese
1/2 cup heavy cream
1/4 cup chicken broth
1 cup crushed pecans
3 TBS Butter

Peel turnips and shred with a cheese grater into hash brown shapes. Option: soak the turnips in chicken broth overnight. Spread shredded turnips in 9x13" baking dish. Mix onions, cheese, cream cheese, heavy cream, broth and sour cream until completely mixed. Mix in turnips. Melt butter, mix with pecans and sprinkle on top. Bake at 350°F for 30 minutes. (or in crockpot for 10-12 hours). Makes 8 servings.

NUTRITIONAL COMPARISON (per serving):
Using Potatoes = 504 calories, 36.5 carbs, 2.3 fiber, 9.1 protein
Using Turnips = 413 calories, 16.5 carbs, 1.5 fiber, 9.1 protein

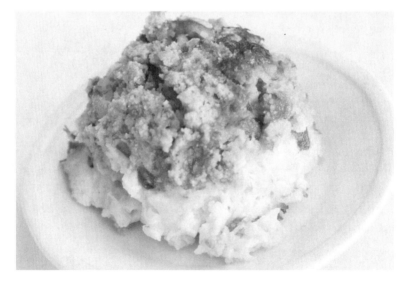

FAUX-TATO SALAD

2 lbs turnips, halved
2 tsp Celtic sea salt
2 TBS beef broth
6 TBS Spectrum organic
mayonnaise
2 TBS sour cream
4 tsp Dijon-style mustard
2 dashes ground celery seed
1 hard-cooked egg
2 TBS finely minced onion
2 TBS finely minced celery
4 tsp finely minced green pepper
4 TBS minced parsley
Salt and freshly ground pepper to taste

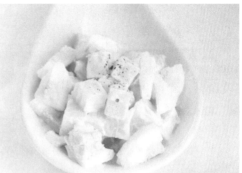

Peel the turnips and place in water to cover. Add salt, bring to a boil, lower flame, and cook 20 to 25 minutes until turnips test done with a fork. Remove turnips from the water and dry on paper towels, then cut in small cubes. Toss turnips with broth while still warm.

Combine mayonnaise, sour cream, mustard, and celery seed. When the turnips have stood in the broth 10 minutes, add sour cream-mayonnaise mixture, and toss lightly. Dice the hard-cooked egg and add along with the onion, celery, green pepper, and parsley. Lightly toss again. Add salt and pepper to taste. Chill briefly and serve. Serves 8 with 7.4g carbs per serving.

NUTRITIONAL COMPARISON (per cup)
Potato = 116 calories, 28 carbs, 4 fiber
Turnips = 36 calories, 8 carbs, 2 fiber

BACON, EGG, AVOCADO AND TOMATO SALAD

1 ripe avocado, chopped into chunks
2 boiled eggs, chopped into chunks
1 medium-sized tomato, chopped
Juice from one lemon wedge
2-4 cooked pieces of bacon, crumbled
Salt and pepper to taste

Mix all ingredients together, stirring not too much, but just enough to make some of the avocado and egg into mush. Makes 4 servings.

Nutritional Information (per serving) = 129 calories, 6 carbs, 3.5 fiber

CALIFORNIA SALAD

1 large tomato, cubed
2 large avocado, cubed
1 cup mozzarella cheese, cubed
1/4 tsp Celtic sea salt
3 TBS balsamic vinegar

Toss together in a large bowl and enjoy! How simple is that?! Makes 8 servings.

Nutritional Information (per serving) = 133 calories, 5.4 carbs, 3.2 fiber

TWICE-BAKED CAULIFLOWER

1 large head cauliflower
4 oz. cream cheese
2 T butter
1/4 cup minced scallions or green onions
1/4 cup freshly grated parmesan cheese
6 slices nitrate free bacon, cooked and cut into pieces
1 cup sharp cheddar cheese (Never pre-shredded cheese)
Sour Cream (for topping)

Preheat oven to 350 degrees F. Cut out stem and core from cauliflower, and cut into small pieces. Cook in large pot of boiling water until cauliflower is tender, but not overly soft. Drain well and mash with potato masher, leaving some chunks. Mix in cream cheese, butter, green onion, Parmesan, and 3/4 of the bacon.

Spread evenly in an 8 X 8 inch glass casserole dish. Sprinkle with cheddar cheese and reserved bacon. Bake 30-35 minutes, or until hot and bubbly. Top each serving with a dollop of sour cream. *If you really want to fool your family, pipe this into a hollowed out potato shell! Makes 6 servings.

NUTRITIONAL COMPARISON (Per Cup of Vegetable Only)
Potato = 116 calories, 28 Carbs, 4 fiber
Cauliflower = 28 calories, 3 Carbs, 1 fiber

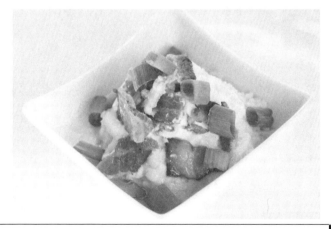

MAIN DISHES

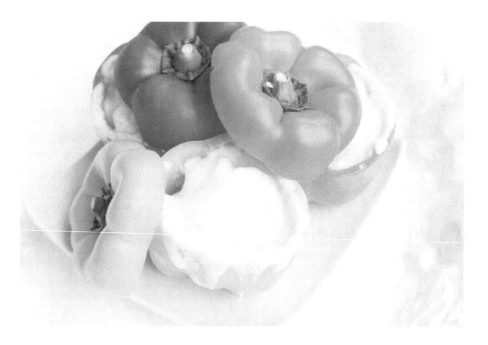

THAI PEANUT "NOODLES"

Noodles:

4 cups zucchini, cut into noodle-like strips

*I used my handy-dandy tool: The Spiral Slicer found on Amazon.com

Peanut Sauce:

2 TBS aged wheat free tamari sauce (fermented soy sauce)

4 TBS natural peanut butter

4 TBS hot water

3 drops Stevia Glycerite

1/4 tsp cayenne pepper

1 1/2 tsp lemon juice

Peanuts for garnish

In a small bowl combine peanut butter and water; mix until a smooth paste forms. Stir in tamari sauce, then the sweetener, cayenne and lemon juice. Mix by hand until well combined and smooth. Mix with the zucchini and enjoy! Option: add chicken or shrimp to make this one hardy meal! Makes 4 servings.

Nutritional Information per serving (1 cup servings) = 72 calories, 5.3 carbs, 1.5 fiber

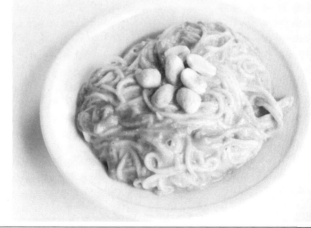

TERIYAKI SAUCE AND SHRIMP FRIED "RICE"

<u>Teriyaki Sauce:</u>

1 2/3 cups organic wheat free Tamari/soy Sauce
1/3 cup macadamia nut oil
1/2 cup Erythritol and 1 tsp Stevia Glycerite
1 clove garlic, minced
2 tsp fresh ginger (I always keep some in the freezer)
3 green onions, minced

Combine all ingredients in a medium size pot. Bring to a boil then
simmer for 30 minutes. Let cool, then strain through a sieve or
cheesecloth. Use as a marinade or just to brush on while grilling. Makes 2
cups
Nutritional information (per TBS)
= 20 calories, 3 carbs, 0.5 grams
fiber

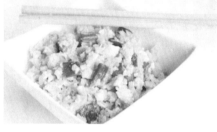

<u>Shrimp "Fried Rice":</u>

2 cups of fresh cauliflower, grated
2 TBS coconut oil or butter
1/3 cup onion, chopped
1 cup broccoli, into bite sized pieces
1 cup green pepper, into bite sized pieces
4 oz shrimp (or other protein like chicken)
2 eggs, beaten
1/4 cup Teriyaki sauce (from above)

Pulse cauliflower using a food processor (or grate it with a cheese grater).
Heat the oil in a pan. Sauté the onions and shrimp for 3-5 minutes over
medium heat, or until shrimp is cooked through, then add the broccoli
and peppers. Stir fry until crisp tender. Add all of the cauliflower; stir
frying for a couple of minutes. Pour in 1/4 of the Teriyaki sauce mixture
and stir fry to coat the cauliflower. When the cauliflower is tender, push
the stir fry to the side of the pan and scramble eggs on the other side,
moving spatula quickly to incorporate eggs with the stir fry. Optional:
add more teriyaki sauce.

4 skinless, boneless chicken breast halves - cut into thin strips
1/2 cup organic Tamari sauce (soy sauce), divided
4 tsp Erythritol, divided
3 TBS rice wine vinegar
2 1/4 cups chicken broth
1 TBS sesame oil
1/2 tsp ground black pepper
12 oz Miracle Noodles
2 TBS coconut oil, divided
2 TBS minced fresh ginger root
1 TBS minced garlic
1/2 tsp guar gum/xanthan gum (natural thickener)
1/2 pound fresh mushrooms, stemmed and sliced
6 green onions, sliced diagonally into 1/2 inch pieces

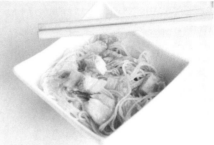

In a medium bowl, combine the chicken with 2 teaspoons of Erythritol, 1 1/2 tablespoons vinegar and 1/4 cup Tamari sauce. Mix this together and coat the chicken well. Cover and let marinate in the refrigerator for at least 1 hour or overnight. In another medium bowl, combine the chicken broth, sesame oil and ground black pepper with the remaining sweetener, vinegar and Tamari sauce. In a separate small bowl, dissolve the thickener with some of this mixture and slowly add to the bulk of the mixture (it will thicken as it sits), stirring well. Set aside. Heat the Miracle noodles according to package directions, drain and set aside. Heat 1 tablespoon of the coconut oil in a wok or large saucepan over high heat until it starts to smoke. Add the chicken and stir-fry for 4 to 5 minutes, or until browned. Transfer this and all juices to a warm plate. Heat the remaining coconut oil in the wok or pan over high heat. Add the ginger, garlic, mushrooms, and green onions, and stir-fry for 30 seconds. Add the reserved sauce mixture and then the chicken. Simmer until the sauce begins to thicken, about 2 minutes. Add the reserved noodles and toss gently, coating everything well with the sauce. Makes 4 servings.

NUTRITIONAL COMPARISON (per serving):
Traditional Lo Mein = 604 calories, 78.9 carbs, 4.5 fiber
"Healthified" Lo Mein = 220 calories, 5.9 carbs, 4.5 fiber

EASY SHRIMP STIR FRY

24 oz frozen salad shrimp
2 TBS coconut oil
2 green onions, chopped
Teriyaki Sauce:
3 TBS Erythritol and 2 drops Stevia Glycerite
2 TBS soy sauce
1 tsp ground ginger
1/2 tsp garlic powder
1/8 tsp Guar Gum (thickener)

Place shrimp in colander and rinse over large bowl under running, cold tap water 1 minute. Allow to soak in water 5 minutes in order to thaw. Drain.
Teriyaki Sauce: In small bowl, combine sweetener, soy sauce, ginger, garlic powder and guar gum. In large skillet in oil, stir-fry shrimp until liquid accumulates in skillet. Pour off liquid. Add green onions. Stir in Teriyaki Sauce and stir-fry until sauce has thickened. Serve immediately.
Helpful Hint: Add green and red peppers and serve over Cauliflower Rice☺. Makes 4 servings.

Nutritional Information per serving = 191 calories, 3.9 g carbs, 0.9g fiber 34.9 g protein, 3 g fat

1 head of cauliflower
1/4 tsp Stevia Glycerite
1 TBS Rice Wine Vinegar
4 TBS Water
2 TBS Rice Mirin (rice wine)
4 Sheets of Nori
6 Spears of Asparagus, cooked
4 pieces of Smoked Salmon
To serve - pickled ginger, soy sauce and wasabi paste

Filling: Pulse the cauliflower in a food processor until it forms small pieces that resembles rice. Mix together the stevia, rice wine vinegar and water. Add to cauliflower. Microwave or stir fry the cauliflower until it is tender. Add the rice mirin and mix well. Set aside to cool (hint: I have made the cauliflower "rice" in advance to be used for an easy side dish for many dinners). To assemble the sushi: Place a nori sheet shiny side down on a sushi rolling mat. Have the shorter side facing you - like a portrait not landscape! Spread a quarter of the filling onto the half of the nori sheet nearest to you, leaving about 1cm gap from the edge (the shortest edge, nearest to you). Lay strips of smoked salmon horizontally across the center of the filling. Lay a single row of asparagus (about 1 1/2 spears) horizontally on top of the salmon. Moisten the far edge of the nori sheet with a little water. Using the sushi mat and your fingers carefully roll the nori sheet up and over the filling. Roll up tightly as possible - when you have made the roll, if you hold the sushi mat around the roll and pull out the bottom edge of the mat it will help to tighten the rolls. Repeat to make 4 rolls. To serve: Wet a sharp serrated knife and cut each roll into 8 portions. Serve with Japanese pickled ginger, soy sauce and wasabi paste.

NUTRITIONAL COMPARISON (per 8 pieces):
Traditional California Roll = 266 calories, 36 carbs, trace fiber
"Healthified" Sushi Roll = 120 calories, 4 carbs, 1.5 fiber

OPEN-FACED PROVOLONE CHICKEN "SANDWICH"

2 Portobello mushrooms, stems removed and chopped
2 chicken breasts
2 TBS tamari sauce (or soy sauce)
2 TBS plus 1 tsp olive oil, divided
1 garlic clove, minced
2 slices provolone cheese
1/4 tsp pepper
2 TBS chicken broth
2 tsp chopped fresh chives

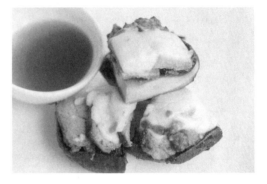

Heat oven to 400 degrees F. Lightly grease medium baking dish; place mushroom caps in dish, gill-side down. Place chicken in shallow dish. Combine Tamari sauce, 2 TBS oil and garlic in small bowl. Brush half the mixture over both sides of mushroom caps. Pour remaining mixture over chicken, turning to coat all sides. Bake mushroom caps 15-20 minutes or until tender but not limp, turning once.

Remove chicken from marinade; reserve marinade. Heat remaining 1 tsp oil in medium skillet over medium-high heat until hot. Cook chicken 4 minutes or until browned on one side. Turn; add mushroom stems to skillet. Top each breast with one cheese slice; sprinkle with pepper. Pour reserved chicken marinade into pan; partially cover and reduce heat to medium low. Cook 3-4 minutes or until cheese melts and chicken is no longer pink in center. Place mushroom caps gill side up on plates; top with chicken mixture. Drizzle with pan juices. (If juices are very thin, increase heat and cook until reduced.) Sprinkle with chives. Makes 2 servings.

NUTRITIONAL COMPARISON (per serving):
Provolone Chicken with bread = 520 calories, 25 carbs, 1 fiber
"Healthified" Chicken with mushroom = 440 calories, 9 carbs, 1.5 fiber

Chicken Strips:
1 tsp coconut oil
1/2 pound skinless, boneless chicken breast halves - cut into strips
1/4 tsp Celtic sea salt
2 tsp butter
1 TBS hot pepper sauce

To Make Strips: Heat oil in a large skillet. Season chicken with salt and sauté over medium high heat, stirring frequently, until lightly browned and cooked through, about 7 to 10 minutes. Remove skillet from heat. Add butter and hot pepper sauce to skillet and swirl until the butter melts and the sauce coats the chicken.

Blue Cheese Mash:
8 cups bite-size cauliflower florets (about 1 head)
4 cloves garlic, crushed and peeled
1/2 cup blue cheese
1 tsp butter
1/2 tsp Celtic sea salt
Freshly ground pepper to taste
Snipped fresh chives for garnish

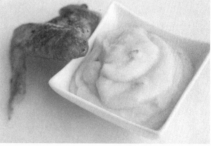

Place cauliflower florets and garlic in a steamer basket over boiling water, cover and steam until very tender, 12 to 15 minutes. (Alternatively, place florets and garlic in a microwave-safe bowl with 1/4 cup water, cover and microwave on High for 3 to 5 minutes.) Place the cooked cauliflower and garlic in a food processor. Add blue cheese, salt and pepper; pulse several times, then process until smooth and creamy. Transfer to a serving bowl. Serve with chicken and enjoy!

NUTRITIONAL COMPARISON:
1 cup Potato = 116 calories, 28 carbs, 4 fiber
1 cup Cauliflower = 28 calories, 3 carbs, 1 fiber

ɔtional, to make a thinner batter)

butter) for frying

...ut ɪlour. Let sit for a minute to thicken up. ...p the batter around the hotdog (I had to use my hands). Add coconut oil or ghee to a skillet on high, once the skillet is hot, place the corndog in the oil and roll around until all sides are cooked OR bake in 350 degree oven for 15 minutes.

NUTRITIONAL COMPARISON (per corndog):
Traditional Corndog = 273 calories, 19.8 carbs, 1 fiber
"Healthified" Corndog = 220 calories, 8 carbs, 4 fiber (before oil absorption)

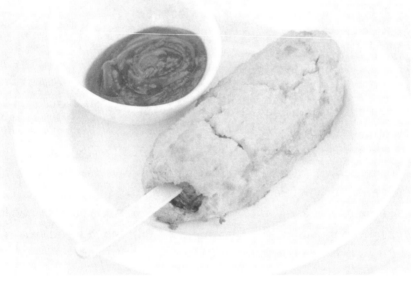

SHRIMP WITH LEMON "RICE" AND CRISPY BASIL

Shrimp:

16 jumbo shrimp (about 1 1/2 pounds), peeled and de-veined

1 TBS ancho chile powder

1 1/2 tsp garlic salt

1 tsp ground coriander

1 tsp dried oregano

1/2 tsp ground cumin

1/2 tsp pepper

1-2 TBS coconut oil or ghee

Lemon Rice:

1 1/2 TBS coconut oil or butter/ghee

1/2 cup finely diced onions

1 clove garlic, minced

4 cups Cauliflower converted into rice

1/4 cup chicken stock

1/4 cup fresh lemon juice

1 1/2 tsp Celtic sea salt plus more to taste

1/4 tsp freshly ground black pepper plus more to taste

1 large zucchini, trimmed, seeded, and diced, optional

Fried Basil:

1 cup coconut oil or ghee

1 large bunch fresh basil, leaves only, well washed and dried

Shrimp: Rinse the shrimp under cold running water. Place the chile powder, garlic salt, coriander, oregano, cumin, and pepper in a mixing bowl and whisk to mix. Add the shrimp and toss to coat. Let the shrimp marinate in the refrigerator, covered, for 30 minutes to 1 hour. Add coconut oil and preheat pan to medium-high heat. When the pan is hot a drop of water will skitter in the pan. When ready to cook, place the marinated shrimp in the hot pan. They will be done after cooking 1 to 3 minutes per side. When done the shrimp will turn pinkish white and will feel firm to the touch.

Lemon Rice: Place cauliflower flowerets in a food processor. Pulse until small pieces of "rice." Heat the oil in a medium saucepan over medium heat. Add the onions and allow them to sweat their liquid for 4 minutes. Add the garlic and sweat for an additional 3 minutes. Stir in the "rice" and zucchini and sauté it for 3 minutes. Add the stock, lemon juice, salt, and pepper. Simmer for 10 minutes, or until the "rice" has absorbed most of the liquid.

Fried Basil: Heat the oil to 350 degrees F on a candy thermometer in a large saucepan over high heat. Standing as far back from the pot as possible and wearing an oven mitt, drop the basil leaves into the hot oil. The oil may bubble and splatter. Fry for about 1 minute, or until the leaves are crisp. Using a slotted spoon, transfer the leaves to a double layer of paper towels to drain. Add as a crispy and flavorful garnish.

NUTRITIONAL COMPARISON:
White Rice = 242 calories, 53 carbs, 0 fiber
Brown Rice = 218 calories, 46 carbs, 4 fiber
Quinoa = 222 calories, 39 carbs, 5 fiber
Wild Rice = 166 calories, 35 carbs, 3 fiber
Cauliflower Rice = 28 calories, 3 carbs, 1 fiber

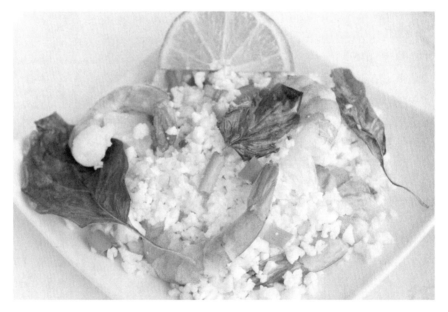

"MACARONI" AND CHEESE

2 jars of Hearts of Palm
Water or chicken broth
Cheese sauce:
1/4 cup butter
3 TBS Cream Cheese
1/4 cup beef/chicken broth
1 cup sharp cheddar cheese,
shredded
1/4 cup Parmesan cheese,
shredded
Sea salt and pepper (to taste)
1/2 cup sharp cheddar (for topping)

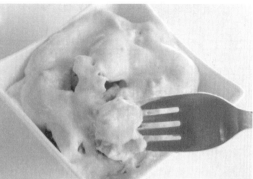

Preheat oven to 375 degrees F. Bring a large pot of chicken broth OR water to a boil. Season the water with salt. Spray the baking dish with olive oil spray. Cut the Hearts of Palm into macaroni noodle shapes. Cook the Hearts of palm in the boiling broth or water until tender, about 5 minutes (You could do this in a microwave too). Drain well and pat between several layers of paper towels to dry. Transfer the hearts of palm to an 8x8 baking dish and set aside. In a saucepan, melt butter over medium heat. Stir in cream cheese and broth. Cook and stir for 2 minutes or until thickened. Reduce heat. Add the cheeses, stirring until cheese is melted. Add salt and pepper to taste. Remove from heat, pour over the veggie, and stir to combine. Top with the additional 1/2 cup cheese and bake until browned and bubbly hot, about 15 minutes. Serves 6.

NUTRITIONAL COMPARISON (per serving):
KRAFT Dinner Mac-n-cheese = 410 calories, 48 carbs, 1 fiber
"Healthified" Mac-n-cheese = 239 calories, 4.9 carbs, 2.7 fiber

1 TBS red wine vinegar

1 tsp Dijon mustard

1 drop of stevia (optional...for sweetness)

1/8 tsp Celtic sea salt

1/8 tsp black pepper

3 TBS extra-virgin olive oil

2 TBS snipped fresh chives

1 pound green beans, trimmed

2 TBS coconut oil or butter

2 cloves garlic, finely chopped

1-1/2 pounds large shrimp, shelled and deveined

1/4 tsp Celtic salt

1/4 tsp black pepper

1 cup cherry tomatoes, halved

1/2 cup crumbled feta cheese

Snipped chives for garnish (optional)

Vinaigrette: In a small bowl, whisk vinegar, mustard, stevia, salt and pepper. Gradually drizzle in the olive oil, whisking continuously until dressing is emulsified. Add chives; set aside.

Green beans and shrimp: Bring a large pot of lightly salted water to a boil. Add beans and simmer for 5 minutes or until crisp-tender. Drain and place in a large bowl. Toss with dressing; set aside.

Heat the 2 tablespoons coconut oil in a large skillet over medium-high heat. Add garlic and shrimp. Season with salt and pepper and cook for about 2 minutes per side or until cooked through. Top with tomatoes and feta. Makes 4 servings.

Nutritional Information (per serving) = 359 calories, 4 carbs, 1 fiber, 24g fat, 32g protein

PORK AND CABBAGE ROLLS

2 pounds of sauerkraut
1 large head green cabbage
2 TBS coconut oil
1 cup finely chopped onions
1/4 tsp of finely chopped garlic
1 lb ground lean pork
2 lightly beaten eggs
2 TBS paprika
1/8 tsp marjoram
1 tsp Celtic sea salt
freshly ground pepper
2 cups tomato sauce (Cantadina Thick and Zesty)
1 cup sour cream

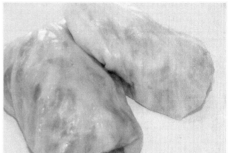

Rinse the sauerkraut in cold water. If needed, soak in cold water 10-20 minutes to reduce sourness. Squeeze dry and set aside. In a large saucepan, bring to a boil enough salted water to cover the cabbage. Add the cabbage, turn the heat to low and simmer 8 minutes. Remove the cabbage and let it drain while it cools enough to handle. Pull off 16 large unbroken leaves and lay them on paper towels to drain and cool further. In a 10-inch skillet, sauté the onions and garlic in coconut oil, until the onions are lightly colored. In a large mixing bowl, combine the pork, eggs, paprika, marjoram, the onion-garlic mixture, salt and a few grindings of black pepper. Mix well with a fork or wooden spoon. Place 2 tablespoons of the stuffing in the center of one of the wilted cabbage leaves and, beginning with the thick end of the leaf, fold over the sides, then roll the whole leaf tightly, as you would a small bundle. Repeat until all the stuffing is gone. Spread the sauerkraut on the bottom of a 5-quart casserole and arrange the cabbage rolls on top of it. Add the water mixed with the tomato puree. Bring the liquid to a boil, then cover the pan tightly and cook over low heat for 1 hour. Transfer the rolls from the casserole to a warm plate. Stir the sour cream into the sauerkraut. Simmer another 5 minutes. Lift the sauerkraut onto a serving platter with a slotted spoon. Arrange the cabbage rolls on the sauerkraut and pour some of the sauce over them. Serve the rest of the sauce in a sauceboat.

BEEF STROGANOFF WITH CABBAGE NOODLES

1 pound ground beef, or thinly sliced beef
Butter, for frying
Half a small onion
LOTS OF MUSHROOMS
1 tsp tomato paste
1 clove crushed garlic
2 cups beef broth
1/2 cup sour cream

Fry the meat and mushrooms in butter on medium/high heat. Remove from the skillet and sauté onions and garlic till onions are tender. Add tomato paste, then the meat. Pour enough beef broth to almost cover the meat. Simmer on low till meat is tender, about 1 1/2 hour... (about 30 minutes for ground beef). Most of the broth should have evaporated.

Taste and add salt and pepper to taste. Add the sour cream and heat through. Serve over Cabbage noodles.

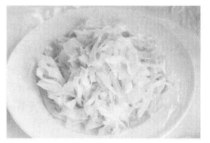

Cabbage Noodles: Slice cabbage into egg noodle widths. Stir fry in butter (or you could boil it in water) for 5-10 minutes or until very tender.

NUTRITIONAL COMPARISON (per cup):
White Pasta = 43 carbs, 5 fiber, 246 calories
Cabbage = 5 carbs, 2 fiber, 22 calories

ROASTED CHICKEN AND PECAN RICE

ROASTED CHICKEN:
1 (3 pound) whole chicken, giblets removed
Celtic sea salt and black pepper
1/2 cup chopped onion
1/2 cup butter, divided
1 stalk celery, leaves removed

Preheat oven to 350 degrees F. Place chicken in a roasting pan, and season generously inside and out with salt and pepper. Place 3 tablespoons butter and the onion in the chicken cavity. Arrange dollops of the remaining butter around the chicken's exterior. Cut the celery into 3 or 4 pieces, and place in the chicken cavity. Bake uncovered 1 hour and 15 minutes in the preheated oven, to a minimum internal temperature of 180 degrees F. Remove from heat, and baste with melted butter and drippings. Cover with aluminum foil, and allow to rest about 30 minutes before serving.

PECAN "RICE:"
3 cups "riced" Cauliflower
2 TBS butter
1/4 cup finely chopped onion
1/2 cup finely chopped pecans
2 TBS minced parsley
1/4 tsp dried basil
1/4 tsp ground ginger
1/4 tsp fresh ground pepper
1/4 tsp Celtic sea salt

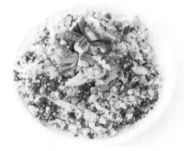

Place cauliflower chunks in a food processor and pulse until it looks like little pieces of rice. In a pan, melt butter and mix in "riced" cauliflower and onions, fry until soft. When cauliflower is done, add pecans, parsley, basil, ginger, pepper and salt. Serve with chicken.

NUTRITIONAL COMPARISON (per cup):
White Rice = 242 calories, 53 carbs, 0 fiber
Cauliflower "Rice" = 28 calories, 3 carbs, 1 fiber

SESAME FISH STICKS

Fish Sticks:
1 1/2 lbs fish fillets
3/4 cup blanched almond flour
Salt and pepper
2 eggs, beaten
1 cup sesame seeds
Coconut oil or expeller pressed Safflower oil
Spicy sweet and sour dipping sauce:
3/4 cup rice vinegar
1/3 cup Erythritol and 1/4 tsp Stevia Glycerite
1/2 tsp red chili pepper flakes
1 tsp Tamari sauce (or soy sauce)
1 large clove garlic, minced

Rinse the fish fillets in cold water. Cut them into approximate 1 inch by 5 inch pieces, following the lines of the fillets. Remove any bones that may remain in the fillets. Lay out 3 separate dishes for dredging, one with almond flour that has salt and pepper sprinkled and mixed in, one with beaten egg, and the last with sesame seeds. Dredge the fish sticks first in almond flour, then in beaten egg, then in sesame seeds. Reserve to a plate. Put enough oil in a large skillet to generously coat the bottom of the pan (about 1/4 cup). Heat the skillet on medium high until the oil is shimmering. Test the oil by dropping a bit of flour into the pan, if it sizzles the pan is ready. Working in batches, add the fish sticks to the pan, leaving enough room around them so that they aren't crowded. Cook for a few minutes on each side, until they are well browned on all sides. Remove the fish sticks to a plate lined with a paper towel. Keep warm in the oven at 160°F while you finish frying the other batches of fish sticks. Add more oil as necessary to the pan to keep the bottom of the pan coated as you fry subsequent batches. To make the dipping sauce, put the sauce ingredients into a small saucepan. Bring to a boil, reduce to a simmer, let cook for 4 minutes, uncovered. Remove from heat and let cool a little before serving. Serves 4-6.

BRAISED BEEF WITH COCONUT RISOTTO

1 grass fed beef stew meat, cut into 2 inch pieces and dried with towel
Salt and freshly ground black pepper
Coconut oil, for searing
2 slices nitrate free bacon, chopped
1 onion, chopped (divided)
1 tsp ginger, chopped
3/4 cup organic wheat-free Tamari (or soy sauce)
4 cups beef stock
2 TBS butter
6 cups cauliflower, pulsed into "rice"
1/2 cups chicken broth
1/2 cup coconut milk
1 tomato, diced
2 sprigs mint, chopped
2 sprigs cilantro, chopped

Preheat the oven to 300 degrees F. Season the beef with salt and pepper on both sides. Heat a large skillet over medium-high heat, and then add enough oil to lightly coat the skillet. Let the oil heat, and then add the beef to the pan, and sear it on all sides until browned. In a Dutch oven or oven-safe pot, cook the bacon slowly over low heat. Add 1/2 the chopped onion, and ginger, and cook for 4 minutes. Add the Tamari sauce and beef stock and boil for 5 minutes. Add the seared beef, and place pot in the oven to braise for 2 1/2 hours. Closer to serving time, make the risotto. Pulse the cauliflower in a food processor until small pieces of "rice." In a medium saucepot, sweat the remaining onion in 2 tablespoons butter for 2 minutes over medium heat. Reduce the heat to low. Add the cauliflower rice, and stir with a wooden spoon to coat it in the butter. Slowly add the chicken broth in 2 equal additions, not adding the second addition until the first has been almost completely absorbed. Stir constantly during the entire process. After all of the chicken broth has been absorbed, add the coconut milk, and then add enough of the braising liquid until the cauliflower is cooked to your taste. Fold in the tomato, and herbs. Serve immediately. Place the "risotto" in the center of a plate and place 2 pieces of beef on top or stir pieces into the "risotto." Makes 6 servings.

NUTRITIONAL COMPARISON (per serving with 4 ounces beef):
Traditional Beef and Risotto = 486 calories, 57.5 carbs, 1.4g fiber
"Healthified" Beef and Risotto = 272 calories, 7.5 carbs, 2.4g fiber

NUTRITIONAL COMPARISON (per cup):
White Rice = 242 calories, 53 carbs, 0 fiber
Brown Rice =218 calories, 46 carbs, 4 fiber
Cauliflower "Rice" = 28 calories, 3 carbs, 1 fiber

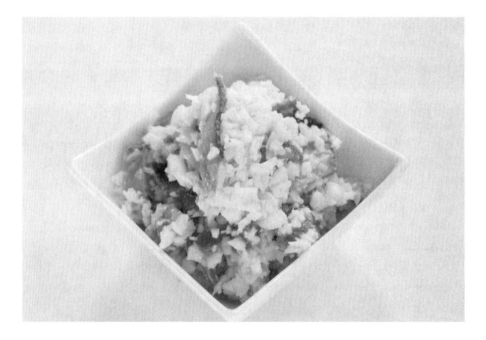

CROCKPOT PHILLY CHEESE PEPPERS

2 TBS coconut oil or butter
1 pound thinly sliced grass fed sirloin steak strips
8 oz. sliced fresh mushrooms
6 green bell peppers
1 medium onion, sliced
6 slices provolone cheese
1(14 oz.) can beef broth
1/2 tsp Celtic sea salt
1/2 tsp ground black pepper
1 garlic clove
2 tsp fish sauce (optional: for "umami")
1/8 tsp red pepper flakes
1/2 cup prepared horseradish (optional)
1/2 cup brown mustard (optional)

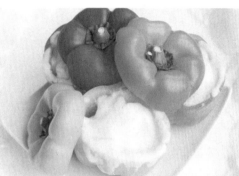

Heat the oil in a large skillet over medium heat. Add the beef, and cook until browned. Add the mushrooms and onion; cook and stir until starting to become tender, about 5 minutes. In a slow cooker, combine the beef broth, salt, pepper, garlic, fish sauce, and red pepper flakes. Transfer the beef and vegetables to the slow cooker, and stir to blend. Cover, and cook on High for 3 to 4 hours, until beef is extremely tender. Preheat the oven to 425 degrees F. Drain the liquid from the slow cooker, and save for dipping. Cut the top of the Green Peppers off, to shape like a bowl. Mix together the horseradish and mustard; spread onto the inside of the peppers. Bake the peppers for 15 minutes or until slightly soft. Remove from oven. Place slices of provolone cheese on insides of the peppers, then fill with the beef and vegetables. Place back in the oven until cheese is melted and serve.

Nutritional Information (per pepper) = 339 Calories; 7.2g Carbohydrate; 2.5g Fiber

BEEF-A-RONI

3 cups eggplant, cut into cubes
4 cups No-Sugar Marinara sauce
1 clove of garlic, minced (optional)
1 1/2 lbs. ground hamburger
1 med. onion, diced
1/2 green pepper, diced
Salt & pepper
1 TBS parsley

Peel and cube the eggplant into 1/2 inch squares. Place in a skillet with marinara and garlic. Simmer for 10 minutes or until the eggplant is soft.

Brown the hamburger, onion and green pepper in skillet. Drain off any excess fat. Add remaining ingredients. Cook over medium-low heat, covered, for 20 minutes. Stir occasionally.

NUTRITIONAL COMPARISON:
1 cup noodles = 246 calories, 46 carbs, 5g fiber
1 cup eggplant = 20 calories, 5 carbs, 3g fiber

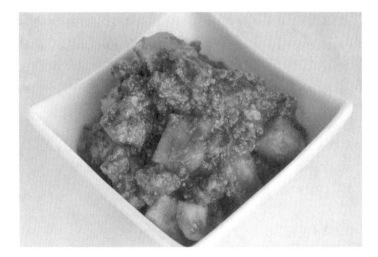

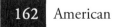

MEATLOAF CORDON BLEU

2 pounds grass fed ground beef
1/2 cup Parmesan cheese, shredded
1/2 cup chopped mushrooms
1 small onion, chopped
2 eggs, beaten
1/8 tsp garlic powder
1 tsp Celtic sea salt
1 tsp pepper
4 oz thinly sliced cooked ham
4 oz provolone cheese, sliced

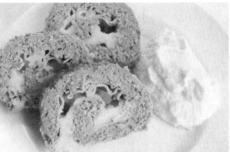

Preheat the oven to 350 degrees F. In a medium bowl, mix together the ground beef, Parmesan, mushrooms, eggs, and onion. Season with garlic powder, salt and pepper. Pat the meat mixture onto a piece of waxed paper, and flatten to 1/2 inch thick (about 8 x 10 rectangle). Lay slices of ham onto the flattened meat, and top with slices of cheese. Pick up the edge of the waxed paper to roll the flattened meat up into a log. Remove waxed paper, seal the ends and seam, and place the loaf into a 9x5 inch loaf pan. Bake for 1 hour and 15 minutes in the preheated oven, or until the loaf is no longer pink inside. Makes 8 servings.

Nutritional Information (per serving) = 376 calories, 4.4g Carbs, 1.7g Fiber, 33.6g Protein

SHRIMP STUFFED EGGPLANT

1 eggplant, halved lengthwise
1/4 cup coconut oil, divided (or butter)
Celtic sea salt and pepper to taste
8 medium shrimp - peeled, deveined and chopped
1/8 cup chopped fresh basil
2 cloves garlic, chopped
1/4 cup broth (chicken or other)
1/2 cup freshly grated Parmesan cheese, divided
Optional: Capers for garnish

Preheat oven to 350 degrees F. Scoop out the flesh of the eggplant, chop, and reserve. Season the shells with salt and pepper; set aside. Heat 1/4 cup coconut oil or butter in a large, deep skillet over medium high heat. Sauté shrimp, basil and garlic until shrimp turns pink, about 1 minute. Stir in the reserved chopped eggplant. Season with salt and pepper. Pour in broth, and cook 5 minutes. Transfer to a large bowl, and mix in 1/4 cup Parmesan cheese. Stuff mixture into eggplant shells, and sprinkle top with remaining Parmesan cheese. Bake in preheated oven for 30 to 40 minutes, or until eggplant is tender. Makes 2 servings.

Nutritional Information (per serving) = 362 calories, 10 carbs, 6 fiber

CHICKEN WINGS WITH BLUE CHEESE DRESSING

3 TBS coconut oil or butter

3 cloves garlic, pressed

2 tsp chili powder, salt and pepper to taste

1 tsp garlic powder

10 chicken wings

Dressing:

2 1/2 oz. blue cheese

3 TBS beef broth

3 TBS sour cream

2 tsp white wine vinegar

2 TBS Olive oil mayonnaise (sauce chapter)

1 to 2 drops Stevia Glycerite

1/8 tsp garlic powder, Celtic sea salt and freshly ground black pepper

Preheat the oven to 375 degrees F. Combine the butter/oil, garlic, chili powder, garlic powder, salt, and pepper in a large bowl. Rub onto the wings with your hands until well coated. Arrange the chicken wings on a baking sheet. Cook the wings in the preheated oven 1 hour, or until crisp and cooked through. Meanwhile, make the dressing. Dressing: In a small bowl, mash blue cheese and broth together with a fork until mixture resembles large-curd cottage cheese. Stir in sour cream, mayonnaise, vinegar, stevia, and garlic powder until well blended. Season with salt and pepper. The dressing makes 4 servings.

NUTRITIONAL COMPARISON (per serving of dressing)

Traditional Blue Cheese Dressing = 241 calories, 1.2 carbs

"Healthified" Blue Cheese Dressing = 104 calories, 1.1 carbs

POTLUCK "RICE" CASSEROLE

1 pound ground grass-fed beef

1 medium green pepper, chopped

1 medium onion, chopped

3 cups cooked Cauliflower "rice"

1 (14.5 oz.) can stewed tomatoes

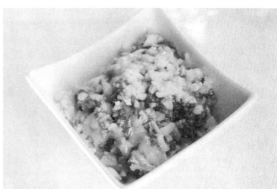

1 can tomato sauce

1 tsp Celtic sea salt

1 tsp chili powder

1 tsp ground mustard

1 tsp dried oregano

1/2 tsp hot pepper sauce

1 cup shredded Cheddar cheese

In a skillet, cook beef, green pepper and onion over medium heat until meat is no longer pink and the vegetables are tender; drain.

Pulse cauliflower in a food processor OR grate with a cheese grater. In another pan, stir-fry the cauliflower "rice" in a TBS of butter until crisp-tender, about 3 minutes. Add the rest of the ingredients, including the beef mixture; mix well.

Transfer to a greased 2-qt. baking dish. Cover and bake at 350 degrees F for 15 minutes. Uncover and sprinkle with cheese. Bake 10 minutes longer or until the cheese is melted.

NUTRITIONAL COMPARISON (per cup):
White Rice = 242 calories, 53 carbs, 0 fiber
Brown Rice =218 calories, 46 carbs, 4 fiber
Cauliflower "Rice" = 28 calories, 3 carbs, 1 fiber

CHILI LIME CHICKEN KABOBS ON "RICE"

3 TBS Coconut oil OR butter
1 1/2 TBS red wine vinegar
1 lime, juiced
1 tsp chili powder
1/2 tsp paprika
1/2 tsp onion powder
1/2 tsp garlic powder
1/2 tsp cayenne pepper
Sea salt and pepper to taste
1 lb chicken breast halves -
cut into 1 1/2 inch pieces
Non-starchy Veggies for grill: Peppers, mushrooms, zucchini

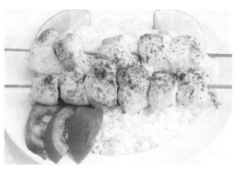

In a small bowl, whisk together the oil, vinegar, and lime juice. Season with chili powder, paprika, onion powder, garlic powder, cayenne pepper, salt, and black pepper. Place the chicken in a shallow baking dish with the sauce, and stir to coat. Cover, and marinate in the refrigerator at least 1 hour. Preheat the grill for medium-high heat. Thread chicken onto skewers, and discard marinade. Lightly oil the grill grate. Grill skewers for 10 to 15 minutes, or until the chicken juices run clear. Serves 4: 227 calories, 3.2 carbs, .9 fiber, 23.9 protein

Serve on top of Cauliflower Rice:
4 cups cauliflower, grated
1 TBS coconut oil OR butter
1/2 crumbled bouillon cube (watch out for MSG and gluten)

Pulse cauliflower in a food processor OR grate with a cheese grater. Add oil to a pan over medium heat. Stir fry cauliflower for 2 to 3 minutes, add the crumbled bouillon cube over the "rice." Cook until just soft and serve with kabobs.
NUTRITIONAL COMPARISON (per cup):
White Rice = 242 calories, 53 carbs, 0 fiber
Cauliflower Rice = 28 calories, 3 carbs, 1 fiber

LEFTOVER TURKEY TETRAZZINI

2 packages Miracle Noodle Linguine
1/2 cup heavy cream
1/2 cup chicken broth
1 egg, beaten
2 cups Cheddar cheese,
freshly grated and divided
1/2 cup grated Parmesan
cheese
1/4 tsp garlic powder
1 tsp poultry seasoning
1/4 tsp fresh ground pepper
3 cups diced leftover turkey
10 oz bag frozen broccoli
Optional additions: mushrooms, peppers, onions, artichokes

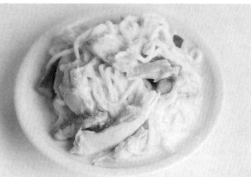

Preheat oven to 400 degrees F. Grease a 9×13″ casserole dish. Rinse Miracle Noodles under running water for a few minutes then pat them totally dry. In a large saucepan heat cream, broth and egg on low. Add 1 1/2 cups Cheddar cheese, Parmesan cheese, poultry seasoning, garlic powder & pepper and stir until melted. Do not boil. Stir in frozen broccoli and turkey. Remove from heat. Meanwhile (if adding), melt butter or coconut oil in a large saucepan over medium heat. Add mushrooms, onion and bell pepper and sauté until tender. Then add to turkey mixture. Place Noodles in the casserole dish. Sprinkle with garlic powder and pepper. Pour turkey mixture evenly over noodles and cover with aluminum foil. Bake for 35 minutes or until hot and bubbly. Remove foil the last 10 minutes and sprinkle with remaining 1/2 cup Cheddar cheese. Bake 10 more minutes. Remove from heat and let sit for 10 minutes before serving. Makes 8 servings.

NUTRITIONAL COMPARISON (per serving):
Traditional Tetrazzini = 504 calories, 39.2 carbs, 2.9 fiber
"Healthified" Tetrazzini = 210 calories, 4 carbs, 2.9 fiber

American

SHEPARD'S PIE

Daikon Mash:
3 cups cubed daikon OR 1 medium head cauliflower
2 cups beef or chicken broth
1 TBS cream cheese, softened
1/4 cup grated Parmesan
1/2 tsp minced garlic
1/8 tsp chicken base or bullion (watch for MSG)
1 egg yolk
1/8 tsp freshly ground pepper
1/2 tsp chopped fresh or dry chives, for garnish
Meat Filling:
1 TBS coconut oil or ghee
1 3/4 pounds ground beef or ground lamb
1 onion, chopped
2 TBS butter
1 tsp guar gum or xanthan gum (thickener)
1 cup beef stock or broth
1 tsp wheat free Tamari (soy sauce)
1 tsp fish sauce (optional: "umami" flavor)
1/2 cup frozen peas (if desired)
1 tsp paprika
2 TBS chopped fresh parsley leaves

To Make Mash: Set a stockpot of broth to boil over high heat. Clean and cut daikon or cauliflower into small pieces. Cook in beef or chicken broth for about 6 minutes, or until well done. Drain well; do not let cool and pat cooked veggie very dry between several layers of paper towels. In a food processor, puree the hot veggie with the cream cheese, Parmesan, garlic, chicken base, yolk and pepper until smooth. Makes 4 servings.

Nutritional Information (per serving) = 153 calories, 8 Carbs, 4g fiber

To Make Filling: While daikons boil, preheat a large skillet over medium high heat. Add oil to hot pan with beef or lamb. Season meat with salt and pepper. Brown and crumble meat for 3 or 4 minutes. If you are using lamb and the pan is fatty, spoon away some of the drippings. Add chopped onion to the meat. Cook veggies with meat 5 minutes, stirring frequently. In a second small skillet over medium heat cook butter and thickener together 2 minutes. Whisk in broth, Tamari and fish sauce. Thicken gravy 1 minute. Add gravy to meat. Preheat broiler to high. Fill a small rectangular casserole with meat and vegetable mixture. Spoon daikon over meat evenly. Top daikon with paprika and broil 6 to 8 inches from the heat until "potatoes" are evenly browned. Top casserole dish with chopped parsley and serve.

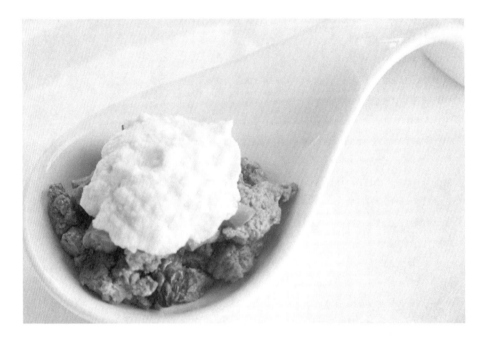

ROLLED TURKEY LOAF AND GREEN BEANS

4 oz. pancetta (or ham) chopped

2 cups chopped portabella mushrooms

2 cups fresh mozzarella cheese, cubed

1/2 cup oil-packed dried tomatoes, drained and chopped

1 egg, lightly beaten

1/2 cup chicken broth

1/2 cup Parmesan cheese, shredded

2 cloves garlic, minced

1 tsp. Italian seasoning, crushed

1 lb. uncooked ground turkey

8 oz. Italian sausage

Fresh oregano

1 recipe Sautéed Green Beans and Onions (recipe below)

Preheat oven to 350 degrees F. In large skillet, cook pancetta until crisp; remove from skillet with slotted spoon and drain on paper towels. Drain all but 1 TBS. drippings from skillet. Cook 2 cups mushrooms in drippings until tender and all liquid has evaporated; cool. For filling, in medium bowl combine pancetta, 2 cups mushrooms, mozzarella, and dried tomatoes; set aside. In large bowl combine egg and chicken broth. Stir in chopped mushrooms, Parmesan cheese, garlic, Italian seasoning, and 1/2 tsp. salt. Stir in turkey and sausage. On heavy-duty foil or parchment, pat meat mixture into a 9x12-inch rectangle. Evenly sprinkle filling on meat mixture. From one long end of foil or parchment, begin rolling the meat mixture jelly-roll-style. Transfer the roll, seam side down, to a 15x10x1-inch baking pan. *See (Roll in Flavor) below. Bake, uncovered, for 1 hour or until an instant-read thermometer inserted into the center of the loaf reads 160 degrees F. Let stand 10 minutes before slicing. Top with oregano. Serve with Sautéed Green Beans and Onions. Makes 8 servings.

<u>Sautéed Green Beans and Onions</u>: in a Dutch oven bring 2 quarts salted water to boiling. Add 2 lb. trimmed fresh green beans. Simmer, covered, for 4 to 5 minutes. Drain, then plunge into ice water to halt cooking.

Drain and pat dry with paper towels. (Beans may be covered and refrigerated up to 24 hours.) In 12-inch large skillet heat 1 TBS. coconut oil and 1 TBS. butter over medium-high heat. Add 1 small thinly sliced red onion and cook until softened and beginning to brown. Add green beans to skillet. Cook and stir for 5 minutes or until heated through. Season to taste with salt and pepper.

*Roll in Flavor: For extra flavor, cheese and veggies are rolled into Rolled Loaf. To shape, place the turkey mixture on parchment or heavy-duty foil. Pat to a 9x12-inch rectangle, and evenly sprinkle with the filling. Beginning at one long side, roll up jelly-roll style, using the parchment to lift and roll. Once rolled, lift using the parchment and transfer to a foil-lined, rimmed baking pan. Use your hands to adjust the loaf seam-side down.

Nutritional Information (per serving) = 402 calories, 10 carbs, 5g fiber, 29g protein, 32g fat

CREOLE "RICE"

4 cups cauliflower, into "rice"
2 links fresh Italian sausage
1 cup chopped onion
5 cloves garlic, minced
1/2 cup diced green pepper
1/2 cup diced sweet red pepper
1 (14.5 oz.) can diced tomatoes, drained
1 TBS lemon juice
1 tsp dried basil
1/2 tsp hot pepper sauce
1/2 tsp poultry seasoning
1/4 tsp chili powder
1/4 tsp pepper
1/8 tsp dried thyme
1 1/4 tsp salt, divided
1 cup diced fully cooked ham
1 cup frozen cooked small shrimp, thawed

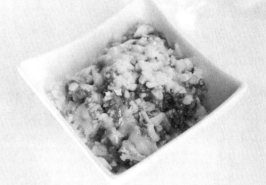

Pulse cauliflower in a food processor OR grate with a cheese grater. Set aside.

In a large skillet, cook sausages. Remove sausages, reserving drippings. When cool enough to handle, cut sausages in half lengthwise, then into 1/4-in. pieces; set aside. Sauté onion, garlic, cauliflower "rice" and peppers in drippings until tender, about 4 minutes. Add the next eight ingredients and 1 teaspoon salt; cook and stir for 5 minutes. Stir in ham, shrimp and sausage; mix lightly. Enjoy!

NUTRITIONAL COMPARISON (per cup):
White Rice = 242 calories, 53 carbs, 0 fiber
Brown Rice =218 calories, 46 carbs, 4 fiber
Cauliflower "Rice" = 28 calories, 3 carbs, 1 fiber

2 medium zucchini
1-2 TBS butter
1 lb. grass fed ground beef
1 med. onion, diced
1 clove garlic, chopped
1/8 tsp Clove
1/8 tsp Ginger
1/8 tsp Chili powder
1/8 tsp Parsley
1/8 tsp Oregano
1/8 tsp Basil
2 cups tomato sauce (Cantadina Thick and Zesty)
5 oz. sharp cheddar cheese, cut into sm. pieces

Prepare zucchini "Noodles": With potato peeler, peel off dark green zucchini skin. With potato peeler, cut zucchini into strips. Rotate zucchini as you go and try to make the strips not too wide. Once you reach the seeds, discard. Place zucchini strips in pan with butter. Sauté over medium-high, stirring to prevent burning. Cook until edges are translucent. Set aside.

Hamburger Instructions: Brown ground beef and drain fat. Add onion, garlic, ginger, and chili powder. Add parsley, basil, oregano, clove. Add tomato sauce and water and stir. Add cheese. Stir to melt cheese. When cheese is completely melted add zucchini noodles. Stir well and serve. Makes 4 servings.

NUTRITIONAL COMPARISON (per cup):
White Pasta = 246 calories, 43 carbs, 0 fiber
Zucchini "noodles" = 20 calories, 4 carbs, 2 fiber

"RISOTTO" WITH BRIE AND ALMONDS

1 head cauliflower (about 6 cups)
3 TBS coconut oil or butter
1/4 cup chicken broth
3 thyme sprigs, plus 1 tsp leaves
5 oz. Brie, rind discarded, cut into small pieces
1/3 cup sliced almonds, toasted

Place cauliflower pieces into a food processor and pulse until small pieces of "rice." Heat butter or oil in a 4-quart heavy saucepan over medium-high heat until foam subsides, then sauté cauliflower with 1/4 teaspoon salt until crisp-tender and golden brown, about 6 minutes. Add thyme leaves and sauté 1 minute. Add broth and briskly simmer, stirring, until broth has been absorbed. Stir in Brie, and salt and pepper to taste. Serve topped with almonds.

NUTRITIONAL COMPARISON (per cup):
White Rice = 242 calories, 53 carbs, 0 fiber
Brown Rice =218 calories, 46 carbs, 4 fiber
Cauliflower "Rice" = 28 calories, 3 carbs, 1 fiber

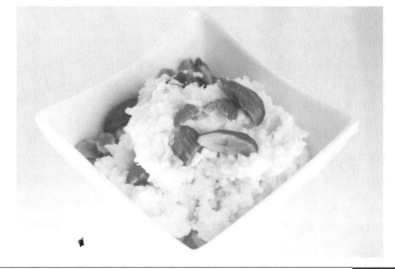

1 head cauliflower (6 cups)
1 TBS coconut oil or butter
1/8 cup onion, diced
1/4 cup grated parmesan
cheese
1 garlic clove, chopped
1/2 cup chicken broth
1/2 cup mascarpone cheese
(or cream cheese)
1/2 cup canned crab
fresh parsley (Garnish)
Celtic sea salt & pepper to taste

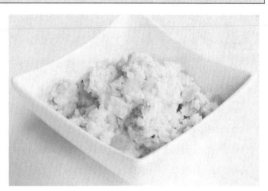

Make the Cauliflower "Rice". Using a food processor grind the fresh cauliflower until it is rice size. Steam or Microwave for 5 Minutes. Use a strainer if necessary to press out any addition liquid. Set Aside.

Sauté the onion and garlic in the oil/butter in a frying pan. Add "rice", salt & pepper, mascarpone and broth. Cook until it starts to reduce approximately 8 min, add parmesan cheese; stir. Toss some fresh chopped Italian Parsley on top before serving. This makes a great hearty main course dish. Makes 4 servings.

NUTRITIONAL COMPARISON:
Traditional Risotto = 226 calories, 40 carbs, 1 fiber, 8.9 protein, 8.2g fat
"Healthified" Risotto = 143 calories, 10.9g Carbs, 4.1g Fiber, 8.9g Protein, 8.2g Fat

THIN AND CRISPY PIZZA CRUST

8 oz. mozzarella cheese, shredded
4 oz. cheddar cheese, shredded
3 eggs
1 tsp garlic powder
1 tsp basil, optional
Toppings of your choice

Mix the cheeses, eggs, garlic powder and basil well. Line a 16-inch pizza pan with parchment paper or nonstick foil. Evenly spread the cheese mixture in the pan, almost to the edge, making it as thin as possible. Bake at 450 degrees F 15-20 minutes until golden brown. I suggest checking it after about 10 minutes. If it's getting very dark on the edges and top, turn the oven down to 400 degrees F and continue baking until brown all over and no longer pale on the bottom. Pat off any excess grease then add your toppings. Keeping the oven rack in the center position, put the pizza under the broiler until the toppings are hot and any cheese you added is melted and bubbly, about 4-5 minutes. Makes 8 servings. Can be frozen

Nutritional Information per serving of Crust only: 176 Calories, 1g carb, trace fiber, 14g fat, 12g protein
Nutritional Information with 1/4 cup pizza sauce, 4 ounces mozzarella cheese, pepperoni, 1/2 cup cooked Italian sausage, 4 ounces mushrooms, 1/4 cup green peppers (per serving) = 271 Calories, 3g carbs, trace fiber, 21g fat, 18g protein

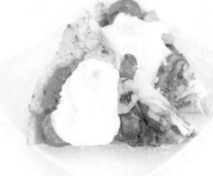

DEEP DISH PIZZA!

Crust:
3 eggs, separated
1/2 tsp cream of tartar
3 oz. Sour Cream
1/2 cup Parmesan cheese, grated
Spices (if desired)

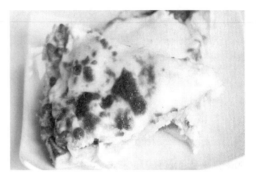

Preheat oven to 375 degrees F.
Separate the eggs and add sour
cream to the yolks. Use a mixer to combine. In a separate bowl, whip egg
whites and cream of tartar until stiff. Then add the Parmesan cheese.
Using a spatula, gradually fold the egg yolk mixture into the white
mixture, being careful not to break down the whites. Spray a lasagna pan
with Olive oil spray and spoon the mixture into it. Bake at 375 degrees F
for 18 minutes. Keep oven shut, and leave for another 5 minutes or until
cool. After it has baked top with your favorite toppings!

Toppings:
No-Sugar Marinara
Chicken sausage
Pepperoni (Trader Joe's)
Mushrooms
Peppers
Mozzarella Cheese

NUTRITIONAL COMPARISON (per slice):
Pizza Hut Deep Dish = 430 calories, 37 carbs, 2 fiber)
"Healthified" Pizza = 157 calories, trace carbs, 0 fiber

PER PIZZA Crust:
1 Little Caesar's 14" Deep Dish Crust = 2,417 calories, 304 carbs
1 "Healthified" pizza crust = 480 calories, 5 carbs, 1 fiber, 37g protein

BBQ CHICKEN LASAGNA

Noodles:
3 cups shredded cheddar cheese
6 eggs, or 12 egg whites
Filling:
2 cups cheddar cheese, shredded
2 tsp liquid smoke
1 tsp Stevia Glycerite
4 cups tomato sauce (Contadina
Thick and Zesty)
4 8-oz. chicken breasts, cooked and shredded
OTHER OPTIONS: mushrooms, peppers, onions...

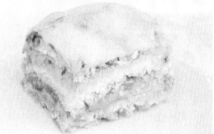

Noodles: Preheat oven to 375 degrees F. Grease 2 large lasagna pans. In a large bowl mix 3 cups of the cheddar with the eggs. Place into prepared lasagna pans into a very thin layer. Bake in oven for 20-30 minutes, or until golden brown...don't under bake though. Remove from heat and set aside to cool. Once cooled, use a pizza cutter to form lasagna "noodles."

Prepare Sauce: Option - use prepared no-sugar added BBQ sauce. OR Place tomato sauce in a large bowl, add the liquid smoke and stevia; mix until combined. Set aside.

Lasagna: Layer the bottom with 1 cup sauce. Layer with 1/2 of the noodles. Layer with 1/2 of the cheese, 1/2 the chicken. Add the rest of the remaining sauce. Top with the noodles, then chicken and top with the cheese. Bake in a 375 degree F oven for 45 minutes, or until bubbly and the cheese is golden brown. Let rest for 10 minutes before serving. Makes 12 servings.

NUTRITIONAL COMPARISON (per serving)
Traditional Lasagna = 427 calories, 36.3 carbs, 4g fiber
"Healthified" Lasagna = 335 calories, 4.6 carbs, 1.3g fiber (using whole eggs)

PORTABELLA PIZZA

2 large portabella mushrooms
1/4 cup canned tomato sauce (Cantadina Thick and Zesty)
1/2 tsp chopped garlic
Dash Italian seasoning
1/2 cup freshly shredded mozzarella cheese
8 slices nitrate free pepperoni
2 TBS sliced black olives

Preheat oven to 400 degrees F. Remove mushroom stems, chop, and set aside. Place mushroom caps on a baking sheet sprayed with nonstick spray. Bake in the oven for 8 minutes. Remove sheet from the oven but leave oven on. Blot excess liquid from mushroom caps and set aside. In a small bowl, combine tomato sauce, garlic, and Italian seasoning. Mix well and equally distribute between mushroom caps; spread until smooth and even. Sprinkle shredded/grated cheese over the saucy layer on each cap. Top with chopped mushroom stems, pepperoni, and olives. Bake in the oven for 8 - 10 minutes, until cheese has melted. Makes 2 servings.

Nutritional Information (per serving) = 118 calories, 7.5g carbs, 1.75g fiber, 11.5g protein, 4.75g fat

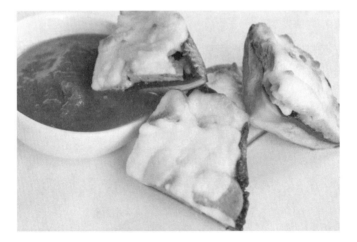

BEAN SPROUT PASTA

2 cups of bean sprouts (remove the roots)
1 clove garlic
1 cup of mushrooms, sliced
1 link of chicken sausage, sliced
Celtic sea salt and pepper to taste
No-sugar marinara sauce (OR Alfredo or pesto)

Bring water in pot to the boil and put the bean sprouts in. I blanch them by putting them in and taking them out of the boiling water immediately. Remove the sprouts and run cold tap water over them. Drain thoroughly. (I stir fried the sprouts this time). Heat some oil in a pan and add the garlic. Brown the garlic and sauté the mushrooms until softened. Cook everything together for about a minute. Top with your favorite sauce and protein.

NUTRITIONAL COMPARISON (per cup):
White Pasta = 246 calories, 43 carbs, 0 fiber
Bean Sprouts = 31 calories, 6 carbs, 2 fiber

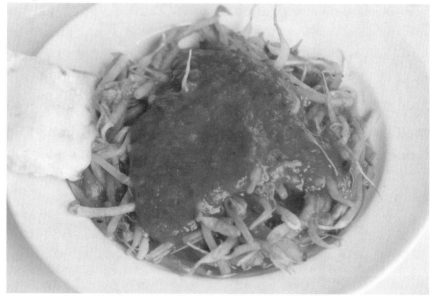

SUMMER SQUASH PASTA & SIMPLE TOMATO SAUCE

2 - 4 zucchini squash
1 14 oz. can diced tomatoes
1 medium fresh tomato
2 cloves of garlic
10 leaves fresh basil
Coconut oil or butter
Celtic sea salt

First run garlic through a garlic press and place into a small bowl or cup. Add 1 tablespoon warm water to the garlic, stir and set aside. Next drain tomatoes and reserve the liquid. Dice fresh tomato into half inch cubes. Chop basil. In a pan heat 2 tablespoon of oil and add the garlic. Cook until fragrant but not brown, about one minute. Add the canned tomatoes and simmer until sauce starts to thicken, about 8 minutes. While the sauce is simmering, peel squash with veggie swirler or with a veggie peeler into long strips. Sauté the squash ribbons in oil on medium heat. Sprinkle with salt and sauté for no more than 2 minutes. Do not allow them to brown or soften. Noodles should be brightly colored and al dente. Remove from pan and set aside. When sauce starts to thicken, add fresh tomatoes and basil. Add some reserved tomato liquid if it becomes too thick to work with. Cook sauce another 3 minutes or so and salt to taste. Toss your sauce with squash noodles and serve immediately.

NUTRITIONAL COMPARISON (per cup):
White Pasta = 246 calories, 43 carbs, 0 fiber
Zucchini "noodles" = 20 calories, 4 carbs, 2 fiber

EASY PIZZA CASSEROLE

1 bag frozen Artichoke hearts
3 links of chicken sausage (Bolinski's Organic)
1 package of sliced mushrooms
1 green pepper
(AND any favorite pizza topping)
4 cups No Sugar Added Marinara Sauce
2 cup freshly shredded mozzarella cheese

Place artichokes in a lasagna pan. Cut up chicken links into 1/4 inch pieces. Top with mushrooms and peppers. Cover the yummy goodness with marinara sauce, top with cheese. Bake at 350 degrees F for 30 minutes and enjoy! Best results are if you let it rest for 15 minutes after baking to let the juices set in.

NUTRITIONAL COMPARISON:
1 cup White Pasta = 246 calories, 43 carbs, 5 fiber
1 cup Artichoke Hearts = 40 calories, 6 carbs, 4 fiber

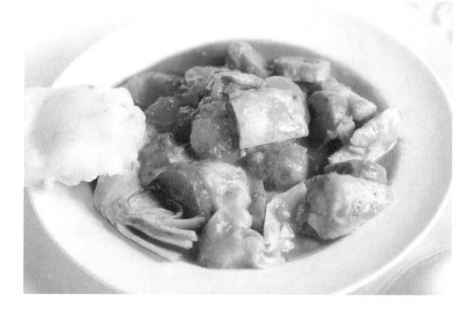

FETTUCCINE WITH TOMATO-BASIL SAUCE

1 pound daikon
1 14.5 oz. can plum tomatoes
3 TBS coconut oil or ghee
1 small onion, finely chopped
2 garlic cloves, minced
1 drop Stevia Glycerite
1 tsp Celtic sea salt
1 TBS fresh basil, chopped
Salt and freshly ground black pepper

With a veggie peeler, peel the outer skin of the daikon and discard.
Continue to peel down the length of the vegetable, removing the daikon
in long, narrow ribbons, which look like fettuccine noodles. Soak the
"noodles" in a bowl of cold salted water for 15 to 20 minutes.
Meanwhile, make the Sauce: Drain tomatoes, reserving half of the juice.
Squeeze tomatoes through your fingers to mash them and combine with
the juice; there will be about 2 cups. In a saucepan, heat oil over
medium-high heat. Add onion and garlic and sauté until soft, about 3
minutes. Add tomatoes and their reserved juice, stevia, and the salt. Boil
vigorously, stirring often, until the sauce thickens, 10 to 15 minutes. Stir
in basil and season with salt and pepper to taste. Drain the "noodles" and
dry them on a kitchen towel. Add them to the sauce and toss gently over
medium heat. Cook just until heated through, about 1 minute. Divide
among plates and enjoy! Makes 3 servings.
NUTRITIONAL COMPARISON:
1 cup White Pasta = 246 calories, 43 carbs, 4 fiber
1 cup of Daikon = 20 calories, 4 carbs, 2g fiber

EGGPLANT PARMESAN

3 eggplant, peeled and thinly sliced
2 eggs, beaten
4 cups almond meal, seasoned with Italian spices and salt
6 cups no-sugar spaghetti sauce, divided
1 (16 oz.) package mozzarella cheese, cut into slices
1/2 cup grated Parmesan cheese, divided
1/2 tsp dried basil

Preheat oven to 350 degrees F. Dip eggplant slices in egg, then in seasoned almond meal. Place in a single layer on a baking sheet. Bake in preheated oven for 5 minutes on each side. In a 9x13 inch baking dish spread spaghetti sauce to cover the bottom. Place a layer of eggplant slices in the sauce. Sprinkle with mozzarella and Parmesan cheeses. Repeat with remaining ingredients, ending with the cheeses. Sprinkle basil on top. Bake in preheated oven for 35 minutes, or until golden brown.

NUTRITIONAL COMPARISON (per 1 large eggplant serving):
Traditional Baked Eggplant Parm = 278 calories, 24 carbs, 8g fiber
"Healthified" Eggplant Parm = 230 calories, 6 carbs, 4 fiber

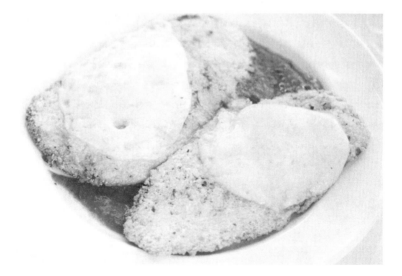

CALZONES!

<u>1 batch dough</u>:
1 large eggplant, (or cauliflower)
1 egg
1 cup shredded mozzarella
<u>Filling</u>:
Pizza sauce (I use Contadina Thick and Zesty Tomato sauce with spices)
Toppings (turkey pepperoni, chicken sausage, olives, mushrooms)
Shredded cheese (GOAT cheese anyone!?)

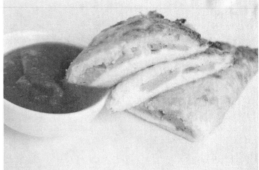

Peel the outside off and cut up eggplant into long lasagna noodle-shaped strips. Place on a sprayed cookie sheet, sprinkle with salt and bake for 15 minutes (to get some moisture out). Preheat oven to 450 degrees F. In a food processor, blend eggplant, egg and cheese. Grease a cookie sheet and form three circles, making sure to press dough out evenly. Bake for 10 minutes, or until the edges are brown. Flip the crusts. Turn oven temperature to 375 degrees F. On one half of each round, spread sauce and top with toppings, careful to stay at least an inch from the edges. Pile high with toppings (again, carefully staying away from edges). Around the edge of the crust, sprinkle a small amount of mozzarella cheese. Fold crust over and press edges together firmly with your fingers by pressing down to the pan, leaving slight indentations. (cheese will melt and help hold crust together as well). Bake for another 30 minutes, or until top is sufficiently golden-brown. Let rest for 5 minutes. Serve with marinara for dipping, or your favorite sauce. Makes 3 calzones.

Per shell (calculate for toppings) = 131 calories, 2 carbs. Trace fiber, 38 protein, 24g fat

CANNELLONI

Celtic Sea salt
1 pound broccoli, washed, florets and stalks chopped
1 pound cauliflower, washed, florets and stalks chopped
Coconut oil or butter
7 cloves garlic, peeled and finely sliced
1 small bunch fresh thyme
1 (1-oz.) can anchovies in oil, drained and chopped, oil reserved
2 to 3 small dried chiles, crumbled
Freshly ground black pepper and salt
2 cups no-sugar tomato sauce
Red wine vinegar
2 cups crème fraiche
7 oz. Parmesan, finely grated
1 large eggplant
1 small bunch fresh basil leaves
7 oz. mozzarella cheese
4 large handfuls arugula leaves, washed and dried
1 lemon

Preheat the oven to 375 degrees F. Bring a large saucepan of salted water (OR I used chicken broth for more flavor) to the boil and drop in the chopped broccoli and cauliflower. Boil for 5 to 6 minutes, until cooked, drain in a colander, reserving the cooking water or broth. Heat a wide saucepan, pour in a couple of TBS of oil and add the garlic. Fry for a few seconds, then add the thyme leaves, anchovies, anchovy oil and chiles and continue frying for a few seconds more before adding the cooked broccoli and cauliflower with around 4 tablespoons of the reserved cooking water. Stir everything together, put a lid on the pan leaving a little gap, and cook slowly for 15 to 20 minutes, stirring regularly - overcooking the vegetables not only intensifies their flavor but gives you the texture that you need for this recipe. Remove the lid for the last 5 minutes to let the moisture evaporate, use a potato masher to crush the vegetables. Take the saucepan off the heat, taste the vegetables and season carefully with salt and pepper. Spread the mixture on a baking sheet to cool. Meanwhile, get yourself another baking dish or roasting pan and pour in the tomato sauce with a pinch of salt and a swig of red wine vinegar. To make a really quick and easy white sauce, mix the crème fraiche with half the Parmesan, a sprinkling of salt and pepper and a little of the reserved cooking water to thin it down.

Peel and cut the eggplant into long thin strips, like a lasagna noodle. Place the filling on the eggplant strip. Roll the eggplant like a cannelloni tube - and place them in a single layer on top of the sauce. Lay the basil leaves over the cannelloni and spoon sauce evenly over the top. Season with black pepper, sprinkle over the remaining Parmesan and mozzarella. Bake in the preheated oven for 30 to 40 minutes, or until golden and bubbling on top. Dress the arugula leaves with a squeeze of lemon juice. Serve the cannelloni with the arugula.

NUTRITIONAL COMPARISON:
1 traditional cannelloni shell = 82 calories, 18 carbs, 1 fiber
1 eggplant cannelloni shell = 30 calories, 4 carbs, 2 fiber

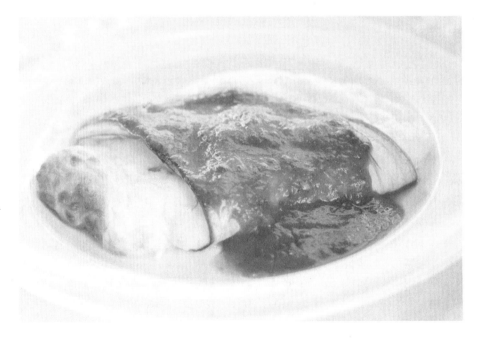

ZUCCHINI ALFREDO

"Pasta":
1 large zucchini (made into 6 cups of "pasta")
Shrimp, crab, scallops...whatever protein you enjoy
Fresh tomatoes, cut into slices
Sauce:
1 stick butter
2 cloves garlic
4 TBS cream cheese
1/3 cup beef broth
1/2 cup Parmesan cheese

Using a veggie swirler shred the zucchini into "noodles." Then set aside.
Place butter in a sauce pan with garlic and cook until light golden brown,
stir constantly, or the butter will burn. Turn to a low heat. Smash up
garlic cloves in the butter. Stir in cream cheese, broth and Parmesan.
Simmer for at least 15 minutes...the flavors open up if you simmer
longer. Serve over zucchini noodles. Top with your favorite protein and
fresh tomatoes. Enjoy!

NUTRITIONAL COMPARISON:
White Pasta = 246 calories, 43 carbs, 0 fiber
Zucchini "noodles" = 20 calories. 4 carbs, 2 fiber

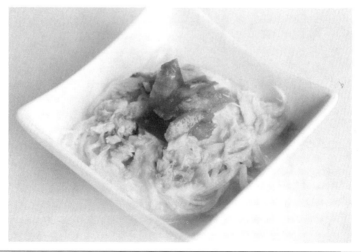

RICOTTA GNOCCHI

1 pound small curd cottage cheese
1/2 pound cheddar cheese
4 eggs beaten
2 TBS flaxseed meal
1 pinch Celtic sea salt, nutmeg and cayenne pepper
1/2 pound butter, melted
1/2 cup grated parmesan cheese

Push cheese through a fine strainer (easy way is with hands) Beat eggs into mixture with electric mixer. Blend in flaxseed meal and seasoning.

Refrigerate for 1 hour. Bring large pot of water to rolling boil. Lower heat to simmer, drop mixture into water by teaspoon full (they will drop to bottom and then rise to the top) Allow gnocchi to simmer on top of water for about 20 minutes. Remove gnocchi carefully with slotted spoon and allow it to drain on absorbent paper.

Melt 1/4 pound butter in large baking dish. Place drained gnocchi in dish, cover with remaining butter and parmesan cheese. Gnocchi may be served immediately or kept warm in low oven or refrigerate and re heat.

Nutritional Information (per serving) = 478 Calories, 3g carbs, 2 fiber, 19g protein

A LIGHER GNOCCHI

2 cups cauliflower, riced
1 pound Ricotta cheese
1 egg
1 oz. real Parmesan, freshly grated
1 tsp Celtic sea salt

Place cauliflower in a food processor and blend until small pieces that resemble rice. Place 2 cups of the "riced" cauliflower in a bowl, and microwave for 3 minutes or until soft (don't add water, cauliflower has enough water to steam itself).

In a large bowl, whip the ricotta to break up the curds. Add the egg and stir until evenly combined. Add the cauliflower, grated cheese and a pinch of salt. Taste and adjust seasonings.

Use a teaspoon to form oval shape gnocchi. Do not let the formed gnocchi touch each other or they'll stick together. Place on a parchment lined cookie sheet. Repeat. Refrigerate two hours or until gnocchi are firm. You can refrigerate overnight. Bake in over for 20 minutes at 375 degrees F or until lightly brown. Serve with favorite low-sugar marina sauce.

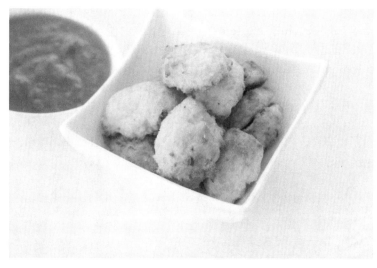

LASAGNA CUPCAKES

24 small cabbage leaves

12 oz. grass fed ground beef

1/4 tsp Celtic sea salt, divided

1/8 tsp black pepper

1 cup chopped onion

1/2 cup chopped mushrooms

1 14.5-oz can crushed tomatoes

1 1/2 tsp chopped garlic, divided

1/2 tsp Italian seasoning

One 10-oz package frozen spinach, thawed and dried

1 1/2 cups ricotta cheese

1 egg

1/8 tsp ground nutmeg

1 1/2 cups freshly shredded mozzarella cheese

Preheat oven to 375 degrees F. Bring a large pot of water to a boil, place whole leaves of cabbage in the water. Boil for 5-7 minutes or until tender. Drain and set aside. Bring a large skillet to medium-high heat on the stove. Add meat, onions, mushrooms, and season with 1/8 tsp salt and pepper. Cook and crumble until no longer pink, about 5 minutes. Reduce heat to low. Add crushed tomatoes, 1 tsp. garlic, and Italian seasoning to the skillet. Stirring occasionally, simmer for 10 minutes. Set aside. Meanwhile, in a bowl, combine spinach, ricotta cheese, egg, nutmeg, remaining 1/8 tsp salt, and remaining 1/2 tsp garlic. Mix well and set aside. Spray a 12-cup muffin pan with nonstick spray. Press a cabbage leaf into the bottom and up along the sides of each cup of the pan. Evenly distribute about half of the spinach-ricotta mixture among the cups, smoothing the surfaces with the back of a spoon. Evenly distribute about half of the meat mixture among the cups, smoothing the surfaces with the back of a spoon. Top each meat layer with 1 TBS mozzarella cheese. Place another cabbage leaf into each cup, lightly pressing it down on the cheese layer and along the sides of the cup, letting the edges fall over the pan. Repeat layering by evenly distributing remaining ricotta mixture and meat mixture among the cups. Top each cup with 1 TBS mozzarella cheese. Bake in the oven until cheese has melted, about 10 minutes. Allow to cool, carefully transfer to a plate, and enjoy! Makes 12 servings.

PER SERVING (1 muffin): 145 calories, 3g carbs, 1.25g fiber

EASY CHICKEN SAUSAGE PASTA

1 head of cabbage (cut into long strips, like noodles)
Garlic and spices for cabbage
2 links of pre-cooked chicken sausage (cut into 1/4 in pieces)
1/2 jar of No Sugar Added Marinara Sauce
1 cup freshly grated Parmesan cheese

Lightly sauté cabbage with 1/2 TBS butter or coconut oil. I added a tsp of garlic and a teaspoon of spices (with NO fillers). Sauté until soft like a noodle. I added pre-cooked chicken sausage, marinara, and fresh cheese. It is an easy AWESOME dinner. I served it with a piece of homemade protein bread.

NUTRITIONAL COMPARISON (per cup):
White Pasta = 246 calories, 43 carbs, 5 fiber
Cabbage "Pasta" = 22 calories, 5 carbs, 2 fiber

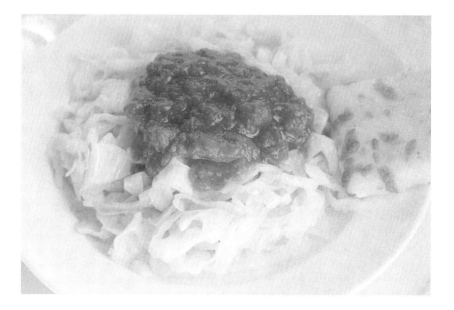

WHITE LASAGNA

Noodles:
1 pound deli shaved chicken breast
Filling:
3/4 cup minced shallots
8 TBS butter
1/2 tsp grated nutmeg
6 TBS cream cheese
3/4 cup chicken stock
2 large eggs, lightly beaten
1/2 tsp Celtic sea salt
1 cup grated Parmigiano-Reggiano, divided
1 serving of "noodles"
OPTIONAL: chicken, mushrooms, or my favorite addition CRAB!

Preheat oven to 350 degrees F with rack in middle. Cook shallots in butter in a heavy medium saucepan over medium heat, stirring occasionally, until tender, about 4 minutes. Add nutmeg, then slowly whisk in cream cheese and stock. Bring to a boil, whisking, then simmer, stirring occasionally, just until sauce lightly coats back of spoon, about 1 minute. Remove from heat and cool to warm, stirring occasionally. Stir in eggs, sea salt, 1/2 teaspoon pepper, and 1/2 cup cheese. Spread about 1 1/4 cups sauce over bottom of an 11- by 8-inch baking dish. Cover with a layer of 3 "noodles", then additional fillings such as crab. Repeat layering 3 more times, then top with remaining sauce and remaining 1/2 cup cheese. Bake, uncovered, until browned, 45 to 55 minutes.

NUTRITIONAL COMPARISON (per cup):
White Flour Noodles = 246 calories, 43 carbs, 5 fiber
"Healthified" Noodles = 84 calories, 2 carb, 0 fiber

CABBAGE LASAGNA

1 pound Italian sausage

3/4 pound grass fed ground beef

1/2 Cup minced onion

2 cloves garlic, crushed

1 (28 oz.) can crushed tomatoes

3 (6.5 oz.) cans tomato sauce (Contadina Thick and Zesty)

1 1/2 tsp dried basil leaves

1/2 tsp fennel seeds

1 tsp Italian seasoning

1 TBS Celtic sea salt, plus 1/2 tsp

1/4 tsp ground black pepper

4 TBS chopped fresh parsley

1 head of cabbage

16 oz. ricotta cheese

1 egg

3/4 lb. mozzarella cheese, sliced

3/4 Cup Parmesan cheese

Boil water in a large pot. Clean cabbage and gently peel leaves. Place in water, boil for 5 minutes or until soft and tender...they won't soften when you cook the lasagna. Remove from water and drain. Preheat oven to 425 degrees F. In a Dutch oven, cook sausage, ground beef, onion, and garlic over medium heat until well browned. Stir in crushed tomatoes and tomato sauce. Season with stevia, basil, fennel seeds, Italian seasoning, 1 tablespoon salt, pepper, and 2 TBS parsley. Simmer, covered, for about 1 1/2 hours, stirring occasionally. In a mixing bowl, combine ricotta cheese with egg, remaining parsley, and 1/2 tsp salt. Preheat oven to 375 degrees F. To assemble, spread 1 1/2 cups of meat sauce in the bottom of a 9x13 inch baking dish. Arrange cabbage noodles lengthwise over meat sauce. Spread with one half of the ricotta cheese mixture. Top with a third of mozzarella cheese slices. Spoon 1 1/2 cups meat sauce over mozzarella, and sprinkle with 1/4 cup Parmesan cheese. Repeat layers, and top with remaining mozzarella and Parmesan cheese. Cover with foil: to prevent sticking, either spray foil with cooking spray, or make sure the foil does not touch the cheese. Bake for 25 minutes. Remove foil, and bake an additional 25 minutes. Cool for 15 minutes before serving.

NUTRITIONAL COMPARISON (per cup):
Traditional Noodles = 246 calories, 43 carbs, 5 fiber
Cabbage "Pasta" = 22 calories, 5 cars, 2 fiber

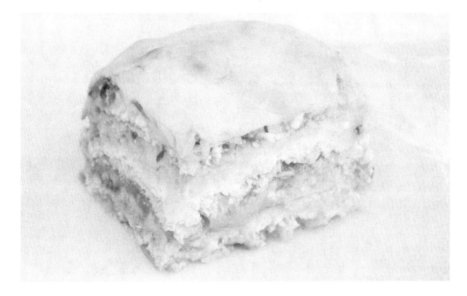

PIZZ-A-RONI

3 cup eggplant, cut into cubes
4 links (Bolinski's) organic pre-cooked Chicken Sausage
1 package nitrate-free pepperoni
1 medium onion, diced
1/2 green pepper, diced
1 cup mushrooms, sliced
Pinch of Celtic sea salt & pepper
1 clove of garlic, minced (optional)
4 cups No-Sugar Marinara sauce

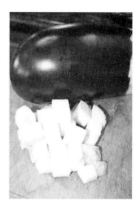

Preheat oven to 350 degrees F. Peel and cube the eggplant into 1/2 inch squares. Place in a skillet with marinara, onion, pepper, mushrooms and garlic. Simmer for 10 minutes or until the eggplant is soft. Slice the chicken sausage into 1/4 inch cubes. In a casserole dish, layer the eggplant mixture, sliced sausage and pepperoni. Add salt, pepper and spices to your liking. Top with cheese and bake for 20 minutes. Enjoy!

NUTRITIONAL COMPARISON:
1 cup noodles = 246 calories, 46 carbs, 5g fiber
1 cup eggplant = 20 calories, 5 carbs, 3g fiber

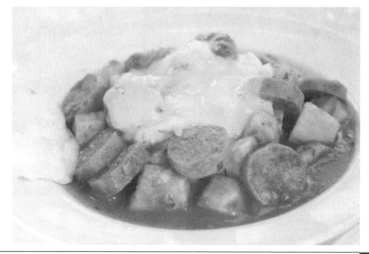

GARDEN SPAGHETTI

2 pounds tomatoes
4 cups zucchini pasta
4 cloves crushed garlic
1 TBS coconut oil or butter
1 TBS tomato paste
Celtic sea salt to taste
1 TBS chopped fresh basil
Freshly ground pepper to taste
1/4 cup freshly grated
Parmesan cheese

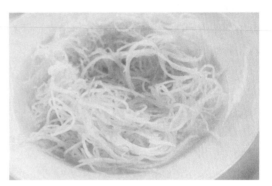

Place tomatoes in a kettle, and cover with cold water. Bring just to the boil. Pour off water, and cover again with cold water. Peel. Cut into small pieces.

Cut zucchini into noodles using a MIU France 90003 Vegetable Julienne Slicer and set aside. (I shaved the peel off first, so it would really look like noodles.)

In a large skillet, sauté the garlic in enough oil to cover the bottom of the pan. The garlic should just become opaque, not brown. Stir in the tomato paste. Immediately stir in the tomatoes, and salt and pepper. Reduce heat, and simmer until the pasta is ready; add the basil. Toss zucchini noodles with a couple of tablespoons of olive oil, and then mix into the sauce. Reduce the heat as low as possible. Keep warm, uncovered, for about 10 minutes when it is ready to serve. Garnish generously with fresh Parmesan cheese. VARIATIONS: Sauté fresh quartered mushrooms with the garlic, or add shrimp, chicken...you name it.

NUTRITIONAL COMPARISON (per cup):
White Pasta = 246 calories, 43 carbs, 5 fiber
Zucchini Pasta = 20 calories, 3 carbs, 1 fiber

SPAGHETTI AND MEATBALLS

2 pounds grass fed ground beef
2 cloves garlic, minced
2 eggs
1 cup freshly grated Romano cheese
1 1/2 TBS Italian seasoning
Celtic sea salt and ground black pepper to taste

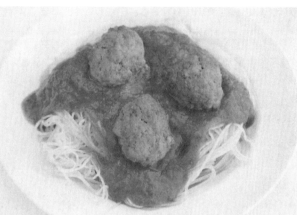

2 cups mushrooms, finely chopped
1 cup beef broth

Preheat oven to 375 degrees F. Combine beef, garlic, eggs, cheese, seasoning, salt and pepper in a large bowl. Blend chopped mushrooms into meat mixture. Slowly add the broth 1/2 cup at a time. The mixture should be very moist but still hold its shape if rolled into meatballs. Shape into meatballs. Arrange in a single layer on a large, shallow baking sheet. Bake meatballs in the preheated oven 35 minutes, turning occasionally, until evenly browned. Serve with Miracle Noodles or Cabbage Noodles and your favorite no-sugar added marinara! Makes 8 servings.

NUTRITIONAL COMPARISON:
Traditional Meatballs = 616 calories, 6.6 carbs, 0.3 fiber
"Healthified" Meatballs = 410 calories, 3 carbs, 2 fiber

NUTRITIONAL COMPARISON (per cup Pasta):
White Pasta = 246 calories, 43 carbs, 5 fiber
Cabbage Pasta = 22 calories, 5 carbs, 2 fiber
Miracle Noodles = 0 calories, 0 carbs, 0 fiber

CHICKEN ENCHILADAS

4 large cabbage leaves
1/2 cup chopped onion
16 oz. raw boneless skinless
chicken breast
1 cup freshly shredded
cheddar cheese, divided
1 cup enchilada sauce,
divided
Optional toppings: sour
cream, scallions

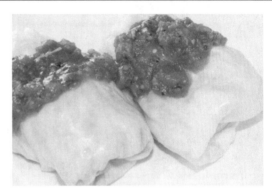

Preheat oven to 400 degrees F. In a pot, boil water and place large leaves of cabbage in the water. Boil for 5-7 minutes or until tender. Spray a baking pan with nonstick spray and set aside. Bring a skillet (with a little coconut oil) to medium-high heat. Add onions and chicken and cook for 4 minutes per side. Cook until chicken is cooked through and onion begins to brown, about 2 more minutes. Set aside. (Option: place frozen chicken breasts and onions in a crockpot before you leave work...they will be tender and cooked when you get home). Once chicken is cool enough to handle, place in a bowl and shred using two forks; one to hold the chicken in place and the other to scrape across the meat. Add 1/2 cup cheese, and 4 TBS enchilada sauce to the bowl with the chicken. Mix well and set aside. Lay cabbage tortillas out flat, and evenly distribute chicken mixture between the centers. Wrap the cabbage tortillas up tightly, and place them in the baking pan with the seam sides down. Pour remaining enchilada sauce over the enchiladas. Bake in the oven until hot, about 10 minutes. Evenly sprinkle remaining cheese over the enchiladas. Bake in the oven until cheese has melted, about 2 more minutes. Place on a plate and top with sour cream and scallions. Serves 4.

NUTRITIONAL COMPARISON (per serving):

Corn Tortilla Enchiladas = 330 calories, 21.5g carbs, 2.25g fiber
Cabbage Tortilla Enchiladas = 253 calories, 8 carbs, 3.5 fiber

TACO PIZZA ON A HEALTHY CRUST

Crust:
1.5 cups raw eggplant OR zucchini, peeled and shredded
2 eggs
2 cups cheddar cheese, freshly grated

Preheat oven to 450 degrees F. Grease cookie sheet. Peel and shred a large eggplant or zucchini. Add egg and cheese, and mix well. Spread the dough evenly onto the pan and bake for 12-15 minutes, or until the crust is cooked. Let cool. Makes one 14 inch crust.

For the Taco Pizza: Layer the pizza with:
Pizza sauce mixed with Salsa
Seasoned ground grass fed beef, cooked
Shredded cheddar
Chopped Tomato
Red Onion
Shredded lettuce

You could also top with guacamole and sour cream if you'd like (change nutritional information if you do). Do not bake with toppings on top. Makes a large, 14" pizza. Serves 8.

Nutritional information (per serving) = 166 calories, 4 carbs, trace fiber, 18g protein, 16g fat

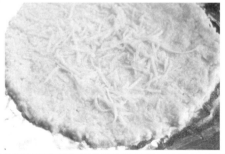

MEXICAN CHICKEN CASSEROLE

1 lb. cooked chicken, diced
1, 14-oz. can sliced mushrooms, drained
4.5 oz. can green chilies
1 TBS chicken bouillon powder
1/2 medium onion
1/2 green pepper
2 tsp olive oil
2 tsp ground cumin
1 tsp chili powder
1/2 tsp black pepper
1/2 tsp onion salt
1/2 tsp garlic powder
1 cup tomato sauce
1 cup water
1/4 cup tomato paste
1 cup grated Cheddar cheese

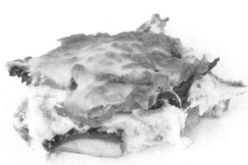

In 9 x 13-inch glass baking dish, combine chicken, mushrooms, green chilies and chicken bouillon powder. In food processor, using S-Blade, process onion and green pepper until finely chopped. In frying pan in oil, stir-fry onion and green pepper until tender. Stir in ground cumin, chili powder, black pepper, onion salt and garlic powder. In small bowl, whisk together tomato sauce, water and tomato paste. Add to vegetables and then add this vegetable mixture to chicken and mushrooms. Combine well. Sprinkle Cheddar cheese over top. Bake in 350 degrees F oven 40 minutes, or until hot and bubbly. Serve with a dollop sour cream, if desired. Makes 6 servings.

Nutritional Information (per serving) = 185.8 calories, 6.5 g carbs, 23.6 g protein, 6.lg fat

SOUTHWESTERN "TABBOULEH"

3 cups Cauliflower
1/4 cup coconut oil or butter
1 cup chopped fresh cilantro
1 cup vertically sliced red onion
3/4 cup diced seeded tomato
1/2 cup sliced green onions
1/2 cup diced yellow bell pepper
1/2 cup chopped peeled avocado
1/4 cup diced peeled cucumber
1/4 cup crumbled queso fresco
2 TBS fresh lemon juice
2 TBS fresh lime juice

2 tsp diced seeded jalapeño
pepper (optional)
3/4 tsp dried oregano
1/4 tsp ground cumin
1/4 tsp ground red pepper
1/4 tsp paprika
1/4 tsp chili powder
1/4 tsp black pepper and salt
1/8 tsp ground allspice
1 garlic clove, minced
Dash of hot pepper sauce

Place cauliflower in a food processor and blend until small pieces of "rice." Place cauliflower rice in a frying pan with oil and stir fry until tender. Add cilantro and remaining ingredients; toss well. Fry for another 3-5 minutes to let the flavors soak into the cauliflower and enjoy! Add your favorite protein and it is a quick meal. Craig liked it more than he thought...he took the leftovers for lunch the next day. Makes 4 servings.

Nutritional Information =140 calories, 4.6g Protein, 9g Carbs, 5.4g Fiber

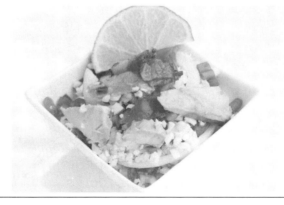

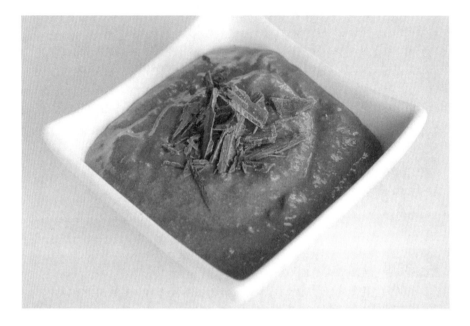

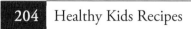

TEDDY GRAHAMS

1/2 cup vanilla whey (Jay Robb brand...no sugar)
3/4 cup almond flour
1/4 tsp baking soda
1/4 tsp Celtic sea salt
1/4 cup butter
2 tsp Erythritol
2 TBS vanilla almond milk OR WATER (to hold dough together)
Cinnamon (for dusting)

Preheat the oven to 325 degrees F. In a medium bowl, stir together the whey, almond flour, baking soda and salt. Cut in the butter using a pastry blender or your fingers until the butter lumps are smaller than peas. Stir in the almond milk and sweetener to form a stiff dough. On parchment paper (lightly sprayed with olive oil spray), roll the dough out to 1/8 inch in thickness. Cut into desired shapes with cookie cutters. Dust with cinnamon. Place cookies 1 inch apart onto cookie sheets. Bake for 7-9 minutes in the preheated oven, until edges are lightly browned. Remove from cookie sheets to cool on wire racks. Makes 24 teddy grahams.

Nutritional Information (per 2 grahams) = 82 calories, 1.5 carbs, 0.75g fiber

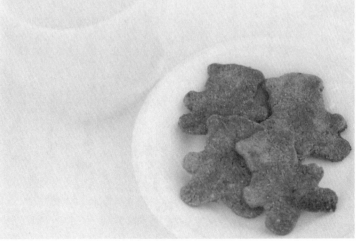

CHEESY DEHYDRATED POPCORN

1 head of cauliflower, broken into 1 inch "florets"
1-2 TBS Butter, melted
1/4 cup walnuts, or sunflower seeds
1/4 cup Parmesan cheese (or nutritional yeast)
1 tsp Celtic sea salt

Place cauliflower "popcorn" pieces into a large Ziploc bag and coat with melted butter. In food processor add nuts (or seeds), Parmesan (or nutritional yeast) and sea salt, process until finely ground. Pour over florets and close top. Shake bag until cauliflower is coated. Place in dehydrator. Dehydrate at 110 degrees F for 6 hours, or until slightly crunchy. If you want it really crunchy, dehydrate for 10 hours. If you fully dehydrate the cauliflower, it will have a week shelf life! What a great camping trip food!

Nutritional yeast has 47 calories, 5 carbs, and 4g fiber, and 8g protein for each heaping 1-1/2 Tablespoon. It also provides you with 1% of the RDA of calcium and 3% RDA of iron. Nutritional yeast is loaded with the B vitamins, and is one of the only vegan sources of vitamin B-12. NUTRITIONAL COMPARISON:
1 cup popcorn = 35 calories, 8 carbs, 1 fiber, 7 effective carbs
1 cup cauliflower = 29 calories, 5 carbs, 3 fiber, 2 effective carbs

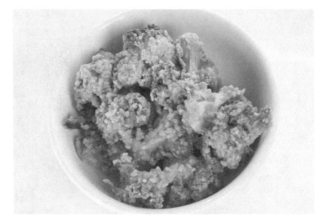

CRISPY CAULIFLOWER POPCORN

1 pound fresh cauliflower
2 TBS butter
4 tsp Mrs. Dash Table Blend

seasoning
Celtic sea salt, to taste

Cut the cauliflower into "popcorn"-size pieces. Put in a large Ziploc bag. Drizzle the melted butter over the cauliflower and sprinkle with Mrs. Dash and a little salt. Close bag and shake until "popcorn" is coated. Spread in a single layer on a baking sheet lined with nonstick foil. Bake at 400 degrees F 50-60 minutes, turning them over every 15 minutes. Bake until dark brown, but not burnt. Taste and add salt, if needed. Makes 4 servings.

Nutritional Information (per serving) = 97 Calories, 7g Carbohydrate, 3g Fiber; 4g Net Carbs, 7g Fat; 3g Protein

PEANUT BUTTER "RICE" CRISPY TREATS

1/2 cup Erythritol and 1/2 tsp Stevia Glycerite
1/2 cup butter
1 cup natural Peanut Butter
1 tsp vanilla
3 cups whey crisps

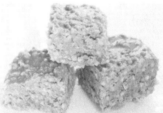

Combine the first 2 ingredients in a saucepan and bring to a rolling boil for 1 1/2 minutes. I then add the other three ingredients and mix until smooth. Place in a greased 9x9 pan, cool and enjoy! Optional: melt a Chocoperfection Bar with 2 TBS almond milk and swirl over the top. Makes 6 servings.

NUTRITIONAL COMPARISON (per serving):
Traditional Rice Krispies = 457 calories, 70 carbs, 2.2 fiber
"Healthified" Rice Crispy Treats = 271 calories, 6 carbs, 2g fiber

GRANOLA BARS

1/3 cup macadamia nuts
1/4 cup pecans
1/4 cup ground almonds
1/4 cup shredded flaked coconut (unsweetened)
1/2 cup vanilla/chocolate whey protein powder
1/8 tsp Celtic sea salt
1 tsp Pure vanilla extract
1/3 cup natural peanut butter (or more)
3 TBS Erythritol and 1 tsp Stevia Glycerite
2 eggs
1/4 cup vanilla almond milk
2 TBS of cocoa powder

Place the pecans, macadamia nuts and almonds in a food processor, and pulse a few times until you have a mix of fine nut powder and some larger nut chunks. Variety in size is good. Add the rest of the dry ingredients. Melt the peanut butter a little bit — 15 seconds in the microwave should do it. Add the eggs, peanut butter, and almond milk. Mix until thoroughly blended. Pour the batter into a greased non-stick or parchment paper-lined 8″ square pan. Smooth it out even so the edges bake evenly. Bake at 350 degrees F for 30 minutes. Fresh out of the oven, cut into rectangles. Store in an airtight container. Makes 12 servings.

NUTRITIONAL COMPARISON (per serving)
Clif Bar = 250 calories, 43 carbs, 5 fiber
"Healthified" Bar = 191 calories,
5 carbs, 2 fiber

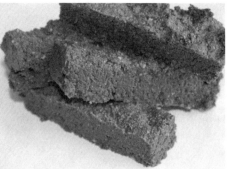

CHOCOLATE "PUDDING"

Have you seen the ingredients in pudding? Yikes! Some have as much sugar as a candy bar. Jell-O pudding contains really high levels of glucose syrup and is also full of refined carbohydrates and artificial additives which can aggravate children's behavioral issues.

3 avocados
6 TBS cocoa powder
1/2 cup chocolate unsweetened almond milk or coconut milk
1/4 cup of Erythritol and 1/4 tsp Stevia Glycerite
Optional: chopped pieces of ChocoPerfection Bar

Whip the almond or coconut milk and the sweetener in a mixing bowl. Peel and pit the avocados. Blend the avocados and cocoa powder in a blender until smooth. Fold the chocolate avocado mix into the coconut and enjoy! Top with pieces of chocolate if desired. Makes 6 servings.

Nutritional Information (per serving) = 153 calories, 5.8 carbs, 3.8 fiber

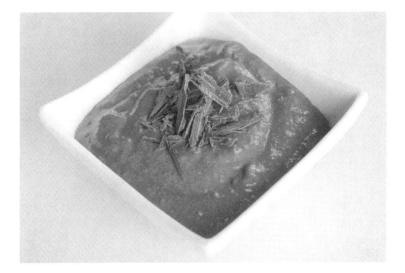

FROZEN YOGURT LOLLIPOPS

1 cup Greek-style natural yogurt
2 drops Stevia Glycerite
1/2 tsp vanilla extract
1 cup fresh or thawed frozen raspberries

Line a baking tray with non-stick baking paper and place in the freezer to chill. Combine the yogurt, sweetener and vanilla in a medium bowl. Place the raspberries in a bowl and use a fork to mash until almost pureed.

Add raspberries to yogurt mixture and gently fold to create a marbled effect.

Spoon 2 TBS of the yogurt mixture onto the prepared tray and spread into an 8cm-diameter circle. Repeat with the remaining yogurt mixture to make another 5 circles. Press a wooden ice-cream stick into the center of each circle. Place in the freezer for 2 hours or until firm. Makes 6 servings.

Nutritional Information (per serving) = 31 calories, 4.5 carbs, 1.5 fiber

Crackers:
1 cup Blanched almond flour
1 cup Parmesan cheese, finely grated
Water (just enough to hold dough together)

Preheat oven to 350 degrees F. Pulse all the ingredients (except for the water) together in a food processor or blender. Add the cold water to the dough, a bit at a time, until the mixture is holding together well enough to work into a ball or two. Roll into 1/2 inch balls. Using your fingers, roll balls back and forth until a stick/log shape. Bake for 20 minutes, or until crackers are browned. The darker, the crispier. Makes 8 servings.

Nutritional Information (per serving) = 136 calories, 3.1 carbs, 1.5 fiber

Cheese Dip:
2 oz. cream cheese
2 oz. sharp (white) cheddar
2 TBS beef broth

Place in a sauce pan and warm on low until melted. Remove from heat and cool. (You could do this in the microwave). This will thicken up as it sets. Makes 4 servings.

Nutritional Information (per serving of dip) = 100 calories, trace carbs

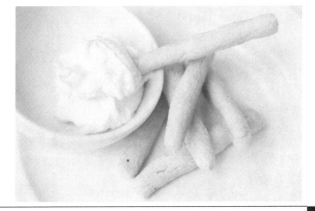

"GOLDFISH" CRACKERS

1 1/2 cups finely shredded cheddar cheese
1 1/2 cups almond flour
1/4 tsp Celtic sea salt
1/2 tsp garlic powder
About 3 TBS cold water to hold the dough together

Preheat oven to 350 degrees F. Pulse all the ingredients (except for the water) together in a food processor or blender. Add the cold water to the dough, a bit at a time, until the mixture is holding together well enough to work into a ball or two. Separate into two balls of dough, and place each ball on a Silpat, parchment paper, or other non-stick surface (which you will transfer to a baking sheet). You can roll it all on one sheet, but I find it easy to do it on two sheets. And two sheets bake more evenly. Roll each dough ball out until flat and about 1/8 to 1/4 inch in thickness. Using a pizza cutter or knife, score the dough into squares, use a Goldfish cookie cutter (found on aStore). Bake for 25 minutes, or until crackers are browned. The darker, the crunchier. Makes 12 servings.

Nutritional Information (per serving) = 136 calories, 3.1 carbs, 1.5 fiber

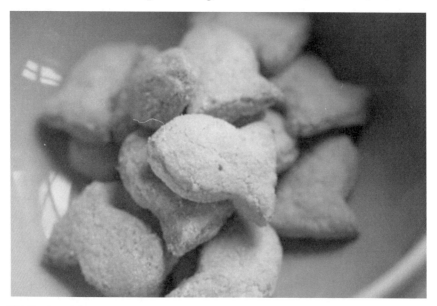

BLUEBERRY BEAUTY

2 oz. cottage cheese
3 oz. plain homemade yogurt
1 to 2 drops Stevia Glycerite
A dash spice mix
1/4 cup fresh organic blueberries, rinsed
2 TBS slivered raw almonds and walnuts

Beat the first 4 ingredients together in a medium bowl. Pour into stemmed dessert glasses. Add blueberries and top with nuts. Enjoy! Makes 1 serving.

Nutritional Information (per serving) = 188 calories, 10.3 carbs, 3.5 fiber

RED, WHITE AND BLUEBERRY SUNDAES

6 large strawberries, sliced
1 cup heavy cream (whipped)
1 cup blueberries
Stevia Glycerite (to taste)
Chopped Nuts (optional)

Divide the strawberries among the glasses. Whip the cream (with stevia) and divide the cream among the four glasses. Layer with crushed nuts. Spoon a layer of blueberries on top and decorate with the U.S flag.

Nutritional Information (per serving) = 136 calories, 8.1 carbs, 1.8 fiber

1/2 cup vanilla whey (Jay Robb...no sugar)

3/4 cup almond flour (doesn't need to be blanched, but helps:)

1/4 tsp baking soda

1/4 tsp Celtic sea salt

1/4 cup butter or coconut oil

1 to 2 drops Stevia Glycerite

2 TBS vanilla almond milk OR water (just enough to hold dough together)

Preheat the oven to 400 degrees F. In a medium bowl, stir together the whey, almond flour, baking soda and salt. Cut in the butter using a pastry blender or your fingers until the butter lumps are smaller than peas. Stir in the almond milk and sweetener to form a stiff dough. On parchment paper (lightly sprayed with olive oil spray), roll the dough out to 1/8 inch in thickness. Cut into desired shapes with cookie cutters. Place cookies 1 inch apart onto cookie sheets. Bake for 5 to 7 minutes in the preheated oven, until edges are lightly browned. Remove from cookie sheets to cool on wire racks. Makes 48 crackers.

Nutritional Information (per 4 crackers) = 82 calories, 1.5 carbs, 0.75g fiber

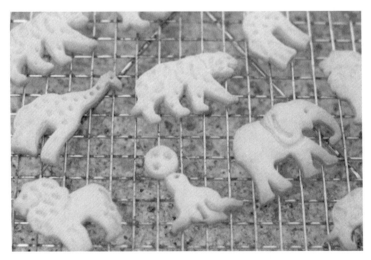

MOCK APPLESAUCE

2 chayote squash
1 TBS butter
1 drop of Stevia Glycerite
1/2 tsp cinnamon or to taste
OPTIONAL: 1 cup Walden Farms Apple Jelly

Cut the squash in half, remove the pit, and peel. Dice and place ingredients in a sauce pan. Turn heat to medium, then cover. They are pretty watery and will basically steam themselves. They should steam for 15 minutes or so. Once soft, remove from heat and puree'. Allow to cool briefly. Makes two servings.

Nutritional Info (per serving) = 11g carbs - 4 g fiber = 7 g net

NO BAKE PROTEIN BALLS

3/4 cup Erythritol and 1/2 tsp Stevia Glycerite
1/2 cup cocoa
1/2 cup butter
2 TBS vanilla or chocolate
almond milk (optional)
1/2 cup natural Peanut Butter
1 tsp vanilla
3 cups chocolate whey crisps

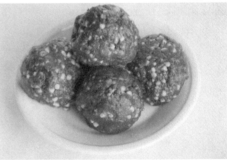

Combine the first 4 ingredients
in a saucepan and bring to a
rolling boil for 1 1/2 minutes. I then add the other three ingredients and drop by tablespoon on wax paper. Let cool and enjoy. Makes 24 servings.

NUTRITIONAL COMPARISON (per serving)
Traditional No Bake Cookies = 152 calories, 19.2 carbs, 1.3 fiber
"Heathified" No Bake Cookies = 109 calories, 3 carbs, 1.3 fiber

DINOSAUR DROPPINGS

1/2 can or 7oz of coconut milk
1 cup almond butter
1 cup 100% cocoa baking chocolate, grated
2 TBS coconut oil
2 TBS egg white or whey protein
2 tsp vanilla
Stevia Glycerite (to taste)
Crushed walnuts (or another nut)

Slowly warm coconut milk in a saucepan on low to medium heat. Add almond butter and stir until smooth. Keep pan on low-medium heat. Add chocolate bar. It will melt easier if you break it into its section. Stir on low-medium heat until smooth. Add coconut oil and once again stir while keeping mixture on low-medium heat. Stir in egg white powder, vanilla and sweetener to taste. Once all stirred and melted, remove from heat. Stir in crushed walnuts (or other nut) and allow mixture to cool enough to handle. You can do this in the freezer or refrigerator to speed it up. After sufficiently cooled, use your hands to roll the mixture into balls. Cool in the freezer or refrigerator. Once cooled and hardened…enjoy! Store in refrigerator. Makes 48 balls.

Nutritional Information (per serving) = 62 calories, 2.1 carbs, 0.75 fiber

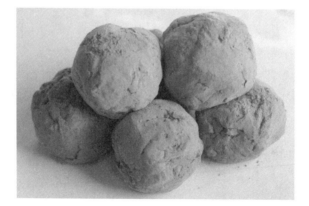

NO-BAKE CHOCOLATE COCONUT ENERGY BARS

1 cup raw sunflower seeds
1 cup raw pecans
4 TBS Coconut Oil
1/2 cup coconut flour
4 drops Stevia Glycerite
1/2 cup raw sunflower seeds
2 TBS almond butter
1 TBS vanilla extract
<u>Chocolate Topping:</u>
4 TBS coconut oil
8 TBS cocoa powder
2-3 TBS Erythritol
Dried, shredded unsweetened coconut

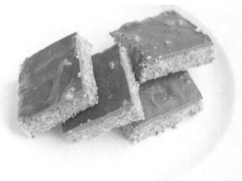

Grind up 1 cup of sunflower seeds and the cup of pecans in food processor or coffee grinder and pour into bowl. Add coconut oil, coconut flour, sweetener, almond butter, vanilla flavoring, 1/2 cup sunflower seeds and mix all together. Pour into square casserole dish and press mixture down firmly.

Sauce: In small saucepan, melt 4 tablespoons coconut oil and mix in cocoa and sweetener until thickened. Pour chocolate sauce on top and sprinkle with shredded coconut. Refrigerate for about 25-35 minutes. Cut up into squares and enjoy! These are also great to pack in your bag for an emergency snack or on a camping trip. Coconut is a stable oil that doesn't require refrigeration. Makes 12 servings.

NUTRITIONAL COMPARISON (per serving)
Power Bar = 240 calories, 45 carbs, 2g fiber
"Healthified" Bar = 278 calories, 10.6 carbs, 5.6g fiber

"APPLES" AND DIP

1 (8 oz.) package cream cheese, softened
1 Cup peanut butter
1/4 Cup Erythritol and 1/4 tsp Stevia Glycerite
1/4 Cup almond milk
1-2 chayote OR jicama, cut into slices

In a mixing bowl, combine the first four ingredients; mix well. Serve with apples. Store in refrigerator.
NUTRITIONAL COMPARISON (per cup)
Apple = 95 calories, 21 carbs, 4g fiber
Jicama = 64 calories, 11 carbs, 6g fiber
Chayote = 22 calories, 5.1 carbs, 2.2g fiber

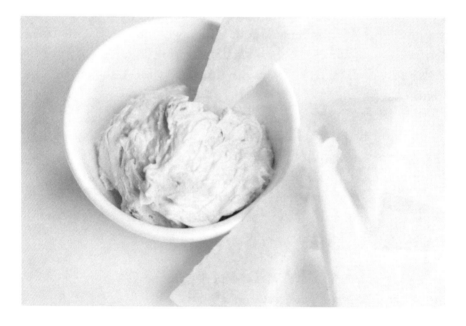

GRAHAM CRACKERS

1/2 cup vanilla whey protein

3/4 cup almond flour

1 tsp cinnamon

1/4 tsp baking soda

1/4 tsp Celtic sea salt

1/4 cup butter or coconut oil

3 to 4 drops Stevia Glycerite (or more to taste)

2 TBS vanilla almond milk (just enough to hold dough together)

Preheat the oven to 400 degrees F. In a medium bowl, stir together the whey, almond flour, cinnamon, baking soda and salt. Cut in the butter using a pastry blender or your fingers until the butter lumps are smaller than peas. Stir in the almond milk and sweetener to form a stiff dough. On parchment paper (lightly greased), roll the dough out to 1/8 inch in thickness. Cut into squares and "score" with a fork (to look like graham crackers). Place squares 1 inch apart onto cookie sheets. Bake for 5 to 7 minutes in the preheated oven, until edges are lightly browned. Remove from cookie sheets to cool on wire racks. Makes 24 crackers. Enjoy with a glass of unsweetened vanilla almond milk.

NUTRITIONAL COMPARISON (per cup)

Skim Milk = 90 calories, 12g sugar

Unsweetened Almond Milk = 40 calories, 0 sugar

Nutritional Information (per 2 crackers) = 82 calories, 1.5 carbs, 0.75g fiber

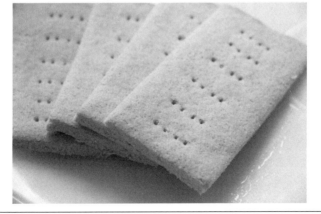

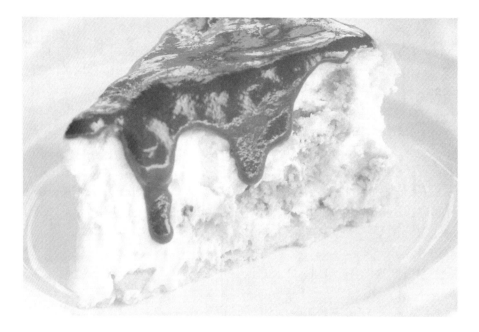

CINNABUN COOKIES

1/2 cup Blanched Almond Flour
1/2 cup vanilla whey protein
1 tsp aluminum free baking powder
3 TBS butter, softened
1 egg

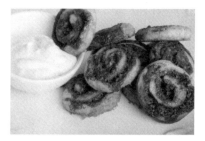

Preheat oven to 325 degrees F. Sift almond flour with whey and baking powder. Add the rest of the ingredients together until you have a smooth dough. Place a sheet of plastic wrap on counter, then spray with olive oil spray. Place dough on greased plastic, push the dough down a bit, and spray with another layer of olive oil. Top with another sheet of plastic wrap. Roll the dough out with a rolling pin until a long rectangle shape (9x12) or so. Remove the top layer of plastic.

Cinnamon filling:
3 TBS Butter, softened
3 TBS Cinnamon
3 TBS Erythritol and 1/4 tsp Stevia Glycerite

Mix all ingredients together and spread evenly over the dough (make sure the top layer of plastic is off.) Roll up dough using the edge of the plastic to make a tight log. Cut into 1/2 inch pieces. Bake for 8 minutes or until baked through (insert a toothpick to check doneness...the toothpick should come out clean).

Frosting:
6 TBS cream cheese, softened
3 TBS butter, softened
2 TBS Erythritol and 1/4 tsp Stevia Glycerite
A little almond milk (to thin it out, if desired)

Mix ingredients together. It will thicken up overnight. Makes 24 cookies.
Nutritional Information (per serving):
Per Cookie with frosting: 80 calories, 0.75 carbs, trace fiber
Per Cookie without frosting: 43 calories, trace carbs, trace fiber

PROTEIN PECAN SANDIES

1 1/2 cup Vanilla Whey (Jay Robb)
1 1/2 cup chopped pecans
1/2 tsp Celtic sea salt
1 tsp pure vanilla extract
1 egg
1/4 cup butter
1/2 cup Erythritol and 1 tsp Stevia Glycerite

Preheat oven to 300 degrees F. Combine the dry ingredients in a bowl. In a separate bowl combine the egg, butter, sweetener and vanilla until smooth. Slowly add the dry ingredients into the egg mixture. Drop spoonfuls on a cookie sheet. Bake on a cookie sheet for 12 minutes or until slightly golden brown. Enjoy! Serves 4 dozen.

NUTRITIONAL COMPARISON (per cookie):
Keebler Pecan Sandies = 90 calories, 9 carbs, 0 fiber, 1 protein
"Healthified" Pecan Sandies = 46 calories, 2.1 carbs, .4 fiber, 5 protein

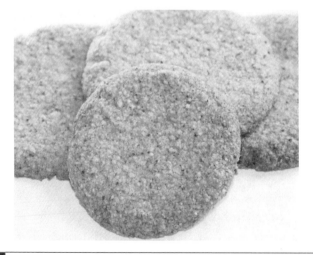

LITTLE DEBBIE OATMEAL CREME PIES

Cookies:
1 cup butter or coconut oil
3/4 cup Erythritol and 1 tsp Stevia Glycerite
1 TBS molasses
1 tsp vanilla
2 eggs
1 1/4 cups blanched
almond flour
1/2 cup vanilla whey
1/2 tsp Celtic sea salt
1 tsp baking soda
1/8 tsp cinnamon
1 1/2 cups crushed
macadamia nuts (to resemble oats)OR vanilla whey crisps

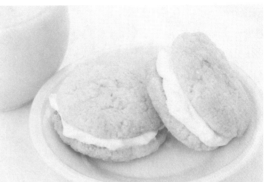

Crème Filling:
2 cups cream cheese, softened
1/2 cup butter, softened
1/4 cup vanilla almond milk OR Walden Farms Marshmallow Fluff
1/3 cup Erythritol and 1 tsp Stevia Glycerite
1/2 tsp vanilla
1/2 tsp Celtic sea salt

Preheat oven to 350 degrees F. In a large bowl, cream together butter, sweeteners, molasses, vanilla, and eggs. In a separate bowl combine the almond flour, whey, salt, baking soda, and cinnamon. Combine the dry ingredients with the wet ingredients. Mix in the macadamia pieces. Drop dough by tablespoonful onto an ungreased baking sheet.
Bake for 10 to 12 minutes, or until cookies are just starting to darken around the edges. They will still appear moist in the center. Be careful not to overcook – when cooled, the cookies should be soft and chewy. While the cookies bake, prepare the filling. Combine the ingredients and mix well with an electric mixer on high speed until fluffy. This mixture will thicken up after it sets. I make this ahead of time and let it sit in my

fridge overnight. Assemble each crème pie by spreading the filling over one side of a cookie (the flat side) and press another cookie on top, making a sandwich. Repeat for the remaining cookies and filling. Makes 1 dozen Large crème pies.

Nutritional Comparison:
Store Bought Little Debbie: 310 calories, 49 carbs, 1 fiber!
"Healthified" Crème Pie: 308 calories, 4.3 carbs, 1.5 fiber (using whey crisps)

YUMMY PEANUT BUTTER COOKIES

2 TBS ground flax
1 cup chunky natural peanut butter
1/2 cup coarsely chopped peanuts
1 cup Erythritol and 1 tsp Stevia Glycerite
1 tsp baking soda
1 large egg

Set aside 1/4 cup of peanuts. Mix all other ingredients together and place small balls on greased cookie sheets. Sprinkle the remaining 1/4 cup peanuts on top of all cookies. Bake at 350 degrees F for 10 minutes. Makes 24 servings.

NUTRITIONAL COMPARISON (per serving):
Betty Crocker Recipe = 110 calories, 12 carbs, 0 fiber, 2 protein
"Healthified" Cookies = 87 calories, 2.7 carbs, 1.1g fiber, 5g protein

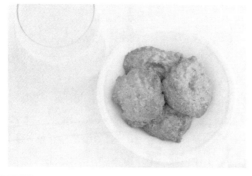

NUTELLA

2 cups raw hazelnuts
1/2 cup unsweetened cocoa powder
1/2 cup Erythritol and 1 tsp Stevia Glycerite
1/2 tsp Pure vanilla
1/8 tsp Celtic sea salt
3 TBS hazelnut oil (could use other oil like coconut)

Heat the oven to 400 degrees F. Spread the hazelnuts evenly over a cookie sheet and roast until they darken and become aromatic, about 10 minutes. Transfer the hazelnuts to a damp towel and rub to remove the skins. Pulsing the Erythritol in a coffee blender and blending it until a fine powder is an optional step, but it makes a really smooth nutella. In a food processor, grind the hazelnuts to a smooth butter, scraping the sides as needed so they process evenly, about 5 minutes. Add the cocoa, sweetener, vanilla, salt and oil to the food processor and continue to process until well blended, about 1 minute. The finished spread should have the consistency of creamy peanut butter; if it is too dry, process in a little extra hazelnut oil until the desired consistency is achieved. Remove to a container, cover and refrigerate until needed. Allow the spread to come to room temperature before using, as it thickens considerably when refrigerated. It will keep for at least a week. Makes 17 servings.

NUTRITIONAL COMPARISON (per 2 TBS):
Traditional Nutella = 200 calories, 23 carbs, 2 fiber
"Healthified" Nutella = 110 calories, 3.4 carbs, 2 fiber

ALMOND COOKIES

1/2 cup vanilla whey (Jay Robb...no sugar)
3/4 cup almond flour
1/4 tsp baking soda
1/4 tsp Celtic sea salt
1/4 cup butter
3 to 4 drops of Stevia Glycerite
2 TBS vanilla almond milk OR water (just enough to hold dough together)

Preheat the oven to 400 degrees F. In a medium bowl, stir together the whey, almond flour, baking soda and salt. Cut in the butter using a pastry blender or your fingers until the butter lumps are smaller than peas. Stir in the almond milk and sweetener to form a stiff dough. On parchment paper (lightly sprayed with olive oil spray), roll the dough out to 1/8 inch in thickness. Cut into desired shapes with cookie cutters. Place cookies 1 inch apart onto cookie sheets. Bake for 5 to 7 minutes in the preheated oven, until edges are lightly browned. Remove from cookie sheets to cool on wire racks. OPTIONAL: Fill with Homemade Nutella. Makes 24 cookies.

Nutritional Information (per 2 cookies) = 82 calories, 1.5 carbs, 0.75g fiber

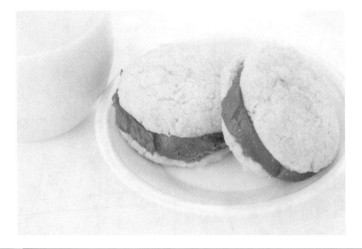

NUTTER BUTTERS

1/2 cup vanilla whey protein
3/4 cup almond flour
1/4 tsp baking soda
1/4 tsp Celtic sea salt
1/4 cup natural peanut butter
1/4 tsp Stevia Glycerite
2 TBS water (to hold dough together)
Filling:
1/2 cup peanut butter
1/2 cup cream cheese
Stevia Glycerite (to taste)

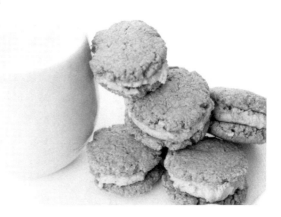

Preheat the oven to 400 degrees F. In a medium bowl, stir together the whey, almond flour, baking soda and salt. Cut in the peanut butter using a pastry blender or your fingers until the butter lumps are smaller than peas. Stir in the water and sweetener to form a stiff dough. On parchment paper (lightly sprayed with olive oil spray), roll the dough out to 1/8 inch in thickness. Cut into desired shapes with cookie cutters. Place cookies 1 inch apart onto cookie sheets. Bake for 5 to 7 minutes in the preheated oven, until edges are lightly browned. Remove from cookie sheets to cool on wire racks. Mix filling ingredients together and use to hold cookies together. Makes 24 mini sandwich cookies.

Nutritional Information (per 2 sandwich cookies) = 178 calories, 3.8 carbs, 1.4g fiber

1/2 cup vanilla whey (Jay Robb...no sugar)
3/4 cup almond flour
4 TBS cocoa powder
1/4 tsp baking soda
1/4 tsp Celtic sea salt
1/4 cup butter
2 drops of Stevia Glycerite
2 TBS water (just enough to hold dough together)
<u>Filling</u>:
8 oz. cream cheese
2 TBS unsweetened vanilla almond milk
4 drops Stevia Glycerite

Preheat the oven to 350 degrees F. In a medium bowl, stir together the whey, almond flour, cocoa, baking soda and salt. Cut in the butter using a pastry blender or your fingers until the butter lumps are smaller than peas. Stir in the water and sweetener to form a stiff dough. On a cookie sheet, place 1/4 inch balls 2 inches apart. Flatten balls into circles (I used a measuring cup). Bake for 10-12 minutes in the preheated oven, until edges are lightly browned. Cool in oven to crisp up. Mix together the filling ingredients and use to hold two chocolate cookies together. Serve with unsweetened vanilla almond milk! Dip and enjoy:) Makes 24 sandwich cookies.

Nutritional Information (per 2 sandwich cookies) = 148 calories, 2.1 carbs, 0.75g fiber

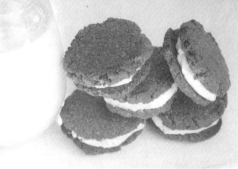

FUDGE ECSTASIES

12 oz. ChocoPerfection chocolate, chopped

1/3 cup Erythritol and 1/2 tsp Stevia Glycerite

2 squares of unsweetened chocolate

2 TBS butter

2 eggs

1 tsp vanilla

1/4 cup peanut flour

1/4 tsp aluminum free baking powder

Dash of salt

1 cup chopped nuts

Preheat oven to 350 degrees F. In a saucepan over medium heat, melt 1 cup of the chips, sweetener, unsweetened chocolate and butter, stirring constantly. Transfer to a large mixer bowl and cool slightly. Add the eggs, vanilla and beat well. Add peanut flour, baking powder and a dash of salt, remaining chips and nuts. Drop dough onto a lightly greased cookie sheet. Bake in oven for 8 - 10 minutes or until edges are firm and surface is cracked and dull. Cool 1 minute on cookie sheet, then remove and cool completely. Makes 36 cookies

NUTRITIONAL COMPARISON (per cookie)
Traditional Cookie with flour and sugar = 102 calories, 11 carbs, 1 fiber
"Healthified" Cookie = 69 calories, 6.7 carbs, 5.3 fiber

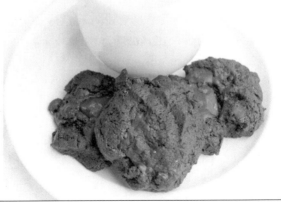

PECAN MACAROONS

2 cups chopped pecans
1/2 cup powdered* Erythritol and 1 tsp Stevia Glycerite
3 large egg whites
3/4 tsp Celtic sea salt
3 TBS Erythritol

*Place 1/2 cup Erythritol in a coffee grinder/food processor and blend until a fine powder. Line 2 baking sheets with parchment paper. Pulse pecans with 1/2 cup powdered Erythritol in a food processor until very finely ground, 2 to 3 minutes, then transfer to a bowl.

Beat egg whites with salt in another bowl with an electric mixer at medium speed until they just hold soft peaks. Add granulated Erythritol, a little at a time, beating, then increase speed to high and continue to beat until whites just hold stiff, glossy peaks. Stir pecan mixture into meringue with a rubber spatula until completely incorporated. (Meringue will deflate.)

Spoon batter into bag, pressing out excess air, and snip off 1 corner of plastic bag to create a 1/4-inch opening. Twist bag firmly just above batter, then pipe peaked mounds of batter (the size of a chocolate kiss) onto lined sheets about 1 1/2 inches apart. Let cookies stand, uncovered, at room temperature until tops are no longer sticky and a light crust forms, 20 to 30 minutes.

Preheat oven to 300 degrees F. Bake cookies for 20-30 minutes or until crisp and edges are just slightly darker. Cool completely on sheets on racks, about 30 minutes. Macaroons keep in an airtight container at room temperature 3 days. Makes 32 cookies.

Nutritional Information (per 2 cookies) = 108 calories, 2 carbs, 1.4 fiber

CHOCOLATE RASPBERRY FRENCH MACAROONS

For macaroons:
2 cups blanched almonds (or blanched almond flour)
1/2 cup powdered* Erythritol and 1 tsp
Stevia Glycerite
3 large egg whites
3/4 tsp Celtic sea salt
3 TBS Erythritol

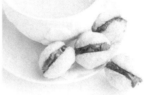

For chocolate raspberry ganache:
3 oz. unsweetened chocolate, chopped
1/3 cup vanilla almond milk
Stevia Glycerite (to taste)
1 TBS coconut oil or butter, softened
1/16 tsp raspberry extract

*Place 1/2 cup Erythritol or erythritol in a coffee grinder/food processor and blend until a fine powder.

Make macaroons: Line 2 baking sheets with parchment paper. Pulse almonds with 1/2 cup powdered Erythritol in a food processor until very finely ground, 2 to 3 minutes, then transfer to a bowl (or use blanched almond flour). In another bowl, beat egg whites with an electric mixer at medium speed until they just hold soft peaks. Add sweetener and salt, a little at a time, beating, then increase speed to high and continue to beat until whites just hold stiff, glossy peaks. Stir almond mixture into meringue with a rubber spatula until completely incorporated. (Meringue will deflate.) Spoon batter into bag, pressing out excess air, and snip off 1 corner of plastic bag to create a 1/4-inch opening. Twist bag firmly just above batter, then pipe peaked mounds of batter (the size of a chocolate kiss) onto lined sheets about 1 1/2 inches apart. Let cookies stand, uncovered, at room temperature until tops are no longer sticky and a light crust forms, 20 to 30 minutes. Preheat oven to 300 degrees F. Bake cookies for 20-30 minutes or until crisp and edges are just slightly darker. Cool completely on sheets on racks, about 30 minutes.

Make ganache while macaroons bake: Melt chocolate with cream in a metal bowl set over a pan of barely simmering water or in top of a double boiler, stirring until smooth. (Bowl should not touch water.) Remove bowl from heat, then add coconut oil or butter and raspberry extract, stirring until butter is melted. Let stand at room temperature until cooled completely and slightly thickened. Carefully peel cookies from parchment (they will be fragile). Sandwich a thin layer of ganache (about 1/2 teaspoon) between flat sides of cookies. Filled macaroons keep in an airtight container at room temperature 3 days. Makes 24 sandwich cookies.

Nutritional Info (per sandwich) = 78 calories, 3 carbs, 1.57 fiber

CHOCOLATE CHIP COOKIES

1 stick butter
1 egg
1 cup Blanched almond flour
1/4 cup Jay Robb vanilla whey
1 tsp baking powder
1 tsp vanilla
1 ChocoPerfection Bar
1/4 cup Erythritol and 2 tsp
Stevia Glycerite

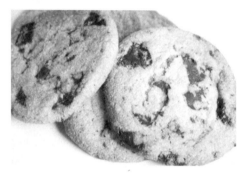

Preheat oven to 350 degrees F. Mix softened butter with sweetener, vanilla and egg. Mix almond flour with baking powder and whey. Slowly mix the wet ingredients with the dry. Add chopped chocolate. Drop spoonfuls onto cookie sheet and bake for 9 minutes at 350 degrees F. Makes 12 cookies.

NUTRITIONAL COMPARISON (per serving):
Traditional Cookie = 211 calories, 24.9 carbs, 1.1fiber, 2.3 protein, 12.4 fat
"Healthified" Cookie =147 calories, 3.3 carbs, 3 fiber, 1.6g protein. 9.5g fat

GINGERBREAD COOKIES

1/4 cup butter or coconut oil
1/4 tsp Stevia Glycerite
1/4 tsp baking soda
1/4 tsp Celtic sea salt
1/4 tsp allspice
1 tsp ground ginger
1/4 tsp ground cloves
1/2 tsp cinnamon
1/2 cup vanilla whey (Jay Robb)
3/4 cup blanched almond flour
1-2 TBS water (to hold dough together)

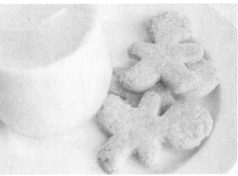

In a large bowl cream the butter and sweetener together until very smooth. Sift the baking soda, spices, salt and whey into the almond flour, then slowly add the almond flour mixture into the butter mixture. Mix until well combined. Form into a tight ball and cool in the fridge to chill. Preheat oven to 325 degrees F. Place the dough onto a non-stick surface (I used parchment paper), then top it with another piece of non-stick surface (again, I used parchment paper) roll the dough out into about 1/4 inch high. Cut the dough with cookie cutters, and place onto a baking sheet. Bake the cookies for 7 minutes, or until light brown. Then turn off the oven and leave the cookies in for an additional 10 minutes, this will create a crispier cookie. Set the cookies out to cool and decorate with cream cheese frosting!

NUTRITIONAL COMPARISON (for 1 large cookie):
Traditional Gingerbread Cookies = 161 calories, 24.4 carbs, 0.6g fiber
"Healthified" Cookies = 101 calories, 2.1 carbs, 1g fiber

WHITE CHOCOLATE SNOWFLAKE COOKIES

1/2 cup vanilla whey (Jay Robb)
3/4 cup almond flour
1/4 tsp baking soda
1/4 tsp Celtic sea salt
1/4 cup butter
4 TBS Erythritol and 1/4 tsp Stevia Glycerite
2 TBS water (to hold dough together)
OPTIONAL: 1/2 tsp nutmeg
1/2 cup La Nouba white chocolate, chopped

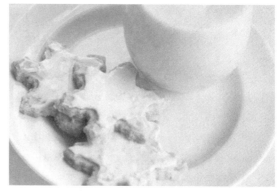

Preheat the oven to 325 degrees F. In a medium bowl, stir together the whey, almond flour, baking soda and salt. Cut in the butter using a pastry blender or your fingers until the butter lumps are smaller than peas. Stir in the water and sweetener to form a stiff dough. On parchment paper (lightly sprayed with coconut oil spray), roll the dough out to 1/8 inch in thickness. Cut into desired shapes with cookie cutters. Dust with nutmeg (if desired). Place cookies 1 inch apart onto cookie sheets. Bake for 7-9 minutes in the preheated oven, until edges are lightly browned. Remove from cookie sheets to cool on wire racks. Meanwhile, melt the white chocolate and 1 tablespoon almond milk (make sure not to burn the chocolate). Stir until smooth. Use white chocolate to frost cookies. Enjoy! Makes 12 servings.

Nutritional Information (per serving) = 92 calories, 2.5 carbs, trace fiber

CHRISTMAS COOKIE CUT OUTS

1/4 cup butter or coconut oil
1/2 cup Erythritol and 1 tsp Stevia Glycerite
1 egg
1 cup blanched almond flour
3/4 cup vanilla whey (Jay Robb)
1/2 tsp Celtic sea salt
1/2 tsp baking soda
1/2 tsp cinnamon
(optional)

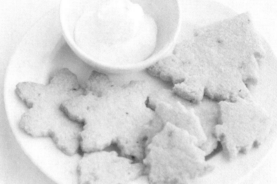

In a large bowl cream the butter, egg and sweetener together until very smooth. Then add the egg and mix until well combined. Sift the baking soda, cinnamon, salt and whey into the almond flour, then slowly add the almond flour mixture into the butter mixture. Mix until well combined. Form into a tight ball and cool in the fridge to chill. Preheat oven to 325 degrees F. Place the dough onto a non-stick surface (I used parchment paper), then top it with another piece of non-stick surface (again, I used parchment paper) roll the dough out into about 1/4 inch high. Cut the dough with Christmas cookie cutters, and place onto a baking sheet. Bake the cookies for 7 minutes, or until light brown. Then turn off the oven and leave the cookies in for an additional 10 minutes, this will create a crispier cookie. Set the cookies out to cool and top with your favorite cream cheese frosting! Makes 2 dozen cutouts.

NUTRITIONAL COMPARISON (for 2 cookies):
Traditional Cookie Cutouts = 161 calories, 24.4 carbs, 0.6g fiber
"Healthified" Cookie Cutouts = 101 calories, 2.1 carbs, 1g fiber

CREME DE PIROULINE

1/2 cup vanilla whey protein
3/4 cup almond flour
1/4 tsp baking soda
1/4 tsp Celtic sea salt
1/4 cup butter or coconut oil
1/4 tsp Stevia Glycerite
1-2 TBS water (to hold dough together)

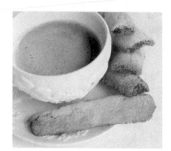

Preheat the oven to 375 degrees F. In a medium bowl, stir together the whey, almond flour, baking soda and salt. Cut in the butter using a pastry blender or your fingers until the butter lumps are smaller than peas. Stir in the water and sweetener to form a stiff dough. On parchment paper (lightly sprayed with olive oil spray), roll the dough out to 1/8 inch in thickness. Cut into desired lengths. Roll around a piece of parchment paper (so there will be a hole for chocolate filling. And place on cookie sheet. Bake for 7 minutes. Leave in oven to cool to crisp up.

CHOCOLATE GLAZE
6 TBS Erythritol, powdered
1/4 tsp Stevia Glycerite (if using erythritol)
4 oz. unsweetened chocolate, chopped
2 TBS unsweetened almond milk (or heavy cream)

Place chopped chocolate, and almond milk in a microwave safe bowl. Heat for 30 seconds, and stir until smooth. Mix in sweetener until smooth. Dip each cookie into the glaze, or drizzle over each cookie. (***For an easy option: Melt a ChocoPerfection bar with 1 TBS almond milk...that is what I did:) Makes 12 cookies.

NUTRITIONAL COMPARISON (per cookie):
Traditional Crème de Pirouline = 150 calories, 19 carbs, 0 fiber
"Healthified" Crème de Pirouline = 92 calories, 2.5 carbs, 1.75g fiber

WHITE CHOCOLATE MACADAMIA BISCOTTI

1/3 cup coconut oil or butter, softened

1/3-1/2 cup Erythritol and 1/2 tsp Stevia Glycerite

2 eggs

1 tsp vanilla extract

2 cups almond flour

2 tsp baking powder

1/2 cup La Nouba white chocolate, chopped

1/4 cup chopped macadamia nuts

1 egg yolk, beaten

1 TBS water

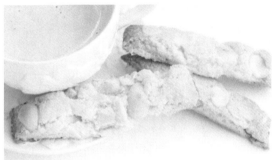

Preheat oven to 375 degrees F. Grease baking sheets, or line with parchment paper. In a large bowl, cream together the butter and sweetener until smooth. Beat in the eggs one at a time, then stir in the vanilla. Combine the almond flour and baking powder; stir into the creamed mixture until well blended. Dough will be stiff, so mix in the last bit by hand. Mix in the white chocolate pieces and macadamia nuts. Divide dough into two equal parts. Shape into 9x2x1 inch loaves. Place onto baking sheet 4 inches apart. Brush with mixture of water and yolk. Bake for 20 to 25 minutes in the preheated oven, or until firm. Cool on baking sheet for 30 minutes. Slice the loaves diagonally into 1 inch slices. Return the slices to the baking sheet, placing them on their sides. Bake for 10 to 15 minutes on each side, or until dry. Serves 30

NUTRITIONAL COMPARISON:
Using white flour and sugar = 71 calories, 10.7 carbs, 0.5 fiber
Using Almond flour = 59 calories, 3.1 carbs, 1.4 fiber

BROWNIE BISCOTTI

1/3 cup butter or coconut oil, softened
1/3 cup Erythritol and 1/2 tsp Stevia Glycerite
2 eggs
1 tsp vanilla extract
1 3/4 cups peanut flour
1/3 cup unsweetened
cocoa powder
2 tsp baking powder
1/2 cup chopped
ChocoPerfection Bar
1 egg yolk, beaten
1 TBS water

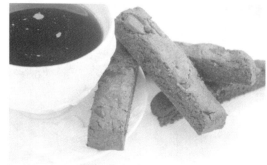

Preheat oven to 375 degrees F. Grease baking sheets, or line with parchment paper. In a large bowl, cream together the butter and sweetener until smooth. Beat in the eggs one at a time, then stir in the vanilla. Combine the peanut flour, cocoa and baking powder; stir into the creamed mixture until well blended. Mix in the chocolate chips. Divide dough into two equal parts. Shape into 9x2x1 inch loaves. Place onto baking sheet 4 inches apart. Brush with mixture of water and yolk. Bake for 20 to 25 minutes in the preheated oven, or until firm. Cool on baking sheet for 30 minutes. Slice the loaves diagonally into 1 inch slices. Return the slices to the baking sheet, placing them on their sides. Bake for 10 to 15 minutes on each side, or until dry. Cool completely and store in an airtight container. Serves 30

NUTRITIONAL COMPARISON:
Using white flour and sugar = 71 calories, 10.7 carbs, 0.5 fiber
Using Peanut flour = 59 calories, 3.1 carbs, 1.4 fiber

EASY ALMOND JOYS

2 TBS coconut oil (melted)
2 TBS unsweetened cocoa
powder
1 TBS almond butter
1 TBS coconut flour
Stevia Glycerite (optional to
taste)

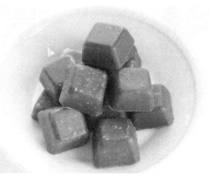

Mix cocoa into the coconut
oil. Then add the almond butter, mix until smooth. Then add the
coconut flour (and stevia if desired). Pour into mini ice cube trays. Freeze
for at least 5-6 minutes and either store in the fridge or freezer. Makes 4
servings.

Nutritional Information Per serving = 88.5 calories, 3.6 carbs, 1.7 fiber

EASY CHOCOLATE PEANUT BUTTER FUDGE

8 oz. unsweetened chocolate squares
1 cup smooth natural peanut butter
3/4 cup Erythritol and 1 tsp Stevia Glycerite
1/2 tsp vanilla
Pinch Celtic sea salt

In a food processor, blend the erythritol until a fine powder. Melt the
chocolate. I like to pour boiling water over it, let it sit for 5 to 6 minutes,
and then pour the water off. That way, you won't burn the chocolate.
Mix in the rest of the ingredients, adjusting sweetener to taste. Spread
into a loaf pan. Cool to room temperature, or you can put it in the
refrigerator. Cut into 18 pieces and serve.

Nutritional Info (per serving) = 146 calories, 6g carbs, 3g fiber, 5g
protein

BUCK-EYE-BALLS

1 1/2 cups creamy natural peanut butter
1/2 cup butter, softened
1 tsp vanilla extract
1 cup Erythritol powdered until fine
6 oz. semi-sweet ChocoPerfection or Simply Lite, chopped
2 TBS unsweetened almond milk

Line a baking sheet with waxed paper; set aside. In a medium bowl, mix peanut butter, butter, vanilla, and confectioners' sugar with hands to form a smooth stiff dough. Shape into balls using 2 teaspoons of dough for each ball. Place on prepared pan, and freeze for at least 30 minutes.

Melt almond milk and chocolate together in a metal bowl over a pan of lightly simmering water. Stir occasionally until smooth, and remove from heat.

Remove balls from freezer. Insert a wooden toothpick into a ball, and dip into melted chocolate. Return to wax paper, chocolate side down, and remove toothpick. Repeat with remaining balls. Refrigerate for 30 minutes to set. Makes 30 servings.

NUTRITIONAL COMPARISON (per serving):
Traditional Buck-Eye Balls = 204 calories, 22.8 carbs, 1.2 fiber
"Healthified" Buck-Eye Balls = 122 calories, 3.7 carbs, 2.15 fiber

PEPPERMINT PATTIES

6 TBS coconut oil
1/3 cup coconut milk
1.5 tsp mint extract, divided
1/3 cup Erythritol and 1/2 tsp Stevia Glycerite
2 (2 oz.) ChocoPerfection chocolate bars or Simply Lite Bars
1/4 tsp Celtic sea salt

Line a muffin pan with pieces of aluminum foil or muffin liners. In a large bowl, mix together the coconut oil, 1/3 cup coconut milk, 1 tsp mint and salt. In a small saucepan, melt the sweetener over medium heat until liquefied. Slowly add the liquefied sweetener into the coconut mixture and mix together thoroughly until you make paste.

Place the mixture into the muffin cups. Place in freezer to leave for 15 minutes or completely cool. Melt chocolate, 1 TBS almond milk, and 1/2 tsp mint and stir until smooth. Dip cooled/frozen coconut mixtures into chocolate, return to wax paper, and place in fridge/freezer to set. Enjoy! Makes 12 servings.

NUTRITIONAL COMPARISON (per serving)
Traditional Peppermint Patty = 165 calories, 34.8 carbs, 0.9g fiber
"Healthified" Peppermint Patty = 99 calories, 3 carbs, 2.4g fiber

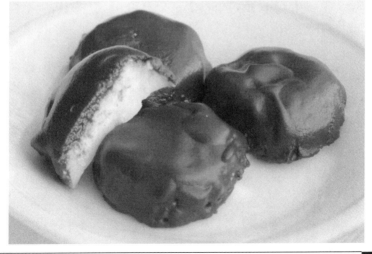

ALMOND BARK

2 TBS heavy cream
2 TBS vanilla almond milk
1/3 cup coconut oil (melted)
1/2 tsp vanilla extract
1 tsp Stevia Glycerite (or to taste)
1/3 cup vanilla whey (Jay Robb)
1/2 tsp guar gum/Xanthum gum (OPTIONAL: thickener)

Mix all ingredients until very smooth. Chill in freezer until set. Top with chopped nuts if desired! Makes 5 servings.

NUTRITIONAL COMPARISON:
Traditional Almond Bark = 210 calories, 20 carbs, 1 fiber
"Healthified" Almond Bark = 93 calories, trace carbs

CHOCOLATE COVERED CHERRIES

2 TBS Heavy cream or coconut milk
2 TBS vanilla almond milk
1/3 cup coconut oil (softened)
1/2 tsp vanilla extract
1 tsp Stevia Glycerite (or to taste)
1/3 cup vanilla Jay Robb whey
12 fresh cherries (or frozen...not maraschino)
2 oz. ChocoPerfection or Simply Lite Bar, chopped fine.

Mix cream, almond milk, coconut oil, vanilla, sweetener, and whey until very smooth. Chill in freezer until set. Form the chilled dough around a cherry. Place back in freezer. Meanwhile, melt the chocolate bar (make sure not to burn or it will get clumpy). Dip chilled wrapped cherries in the chocolate mixture. Set on parchment paper to cool and enjoy! Makes 6 servings.

NUTRITIONAL COMPARISON (per 2 cherries)
Cella's = 120 calories, 19 carbs, 1g fiber
"Healthified" = 84.5 calories, 3.2 carbs, 1.2g fiber

CHOCOLATE ECLAIR DESSERT

3 eggs, separated
3 oz. cream cheese
1/8 tsp cream of tartar
1 tsp Stevia Glycerite

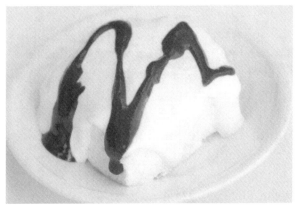

Preheat oven to 300 degrees F. In a bowl, whip egg whites with cream of tartar until peaks are very stiff (about 5 minutes). In separate bowl, blend cream cheese and stevia. Slowly add the cream cheese mixture into the stiff egg whites. (Save yolks for a different recipe). Place in lasagna pan. Bake for 30 minutes. Remove pans from oven and let cool on a cooling rack.

Cream Topping:
8 oz. Cream cheese
1/4 cup unsweetened almond milk
1 tsp Stevia Glycerite (or to taste)

Whip the almond milk, cream cheese and stevia. This mixture will thicken up if you let sit for 4-8 hours. Spread over the puffed éclair.

Chocolate Glaze:
1 CHOCO-Perfection no-sugar added Chocolate Bar
2 TBS vanilla almond milk

In a microwavable bowl, combine ingredients. Microwave for 30 seconds. Stir well. Drizzle onto éclair dessert and let rest on cooling rack until glaze has set. Makes 9 servings.

NUTRITIONAL COMPARISON (per serving):
Traditional Recipe: 370 calories, 63 carbs, 1 fiber
"Healthified" Recipe: 153 calories, 3 carbs, 1.5 fiber

STRAWBERRY CUPCAKES

5 eggs, separated
1/8 tsp cream of tartar
3/4 cup Erythritol and 1 tsp Stevia Glycerite
6 TBS butter (or coconut oil)
1 tsp strawberry extract
1 1/2 cups almond flour
1/2 cup Whey Protein (I used Jay Robb strawberry flavor)
2 tsp baking powder

Preheat oven to 325 degrees F. Whip egg whites with cream of tartar until stiff. In separate bowl, using electric mixer, cream butter with egg yolks until yellow and fluffy. Add vanilla extract and sweetener. Beat until well mixed. Add about 1/3 of the whipped egg whites to the butter/egg yolk mixture and mix lightly. Fold the whole thing into the whipped egg whites and fold lightly. Add 1 cup of the almond flour and fold lightly. Add remaining almond flour, whey protein, and baking powder and fold thoroughly, being careful not to break down whites. Fill paper muffin cups in muffin tin about half full. Bake for about 15 to 20 minutes until cracked on top.

Cream cheese Frosting
3 TBS Butter (I browned the butter first)
3 TBS Cream Cheese
A little vanilla almond milk (to make it spreadable)
1/2 tsp Stevia Glycerite (to taste)

Mix together, top onto cupcakes and
enjoy!

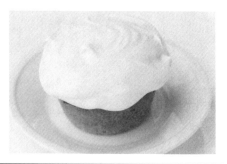

CARAMEL CREAM PUFFS

3 eggs, separated
1/8 tsp cream of tartar
1/2 cup vanilla whey protein
3 oz. cream cheese
1/2 tsp Stevia Glycerite

Preheat oven to 300 degrees F. In a bowl, whip egg whites with cream of tartar until peaks are very stiff (about 5 minutes). Slowly mix in whey protein. In separate bowl, blend cream cheese and stevia. Slowly add the cream cheese mixture into the stiff egg whites. (Save yolks for a different recipe:) Grease a cookie sheet or a medium size muffin tin. Bake for 20 minutes (or until golden brown). Remove pans from oven and let cool on a cooling rack. Once cool, use a knife to cut a small hole in the puffs to insert the cream filling.

Cream Filling:
1 cup heavy cream
1 tsp Stevia Glycerite (or to taste)

Whip the cream until very fluffy, then slowly add in the sweetener to your liking. Place in a large Ziploc bag, cut a small hole in the corner and use to fill the puffs.

Caramel Glaze:
1 cup malitol (other sweeteners won't work)
6 TBS butter
1/2 cup heavy whipping cream

Before you begin, make sure you have everything ready to go - the cream and the butter next to the pan, ready to put in. If you don't work fast, the malitol will burn. You may want to wear oven mitts; the caramelized sugar will be much hotter than boiling water. Heat malitol on moderately high heat in a heavy-bottomed 2-quart or 3-quart saucepan. As it begins to melt, stir vigorously with a whisk or wooden spoon. As soon as it comes to a boil, stop stirring. You can swirl the pan a bit if you want, from this point on. As soon as all of the malitol crystals have melted (the liquid should be dark amber in color), immediately add the butter to the pan. Whisk until the butter has melted. Once the butter has melted, take the pan off the heat. Count to three, then slowly add the cream to the pan and continue to whisk to incorporate. Note than when you add the butter and the cream, the mixture will foam up considerably. Whisk until caramel sauce is smooth. Let cool in the pan for a couple minutes, then pour into a glass mason jar and let sit to cool to room temperature. Store in the refrigerator for up to 2 weeks. Warm before serving over the cream puffs.

Chocolate Glaze:
1 CHOCO-Perfection no-sugar added Chocolate Bar
2 TBS vanilla almond milk

In a microwavable bowl, combine ingredients. Microwave for 30 seconds. Stir well. Drizzle onto éclair dessert and let rest on cooling rack until glaze has set. Makes 24 cream puffs.

Nutritional Comparison (per 2 puffs with 2 TBS caramel sauce):
"Traditional" Recipe: 335 calories, 30 carbs, 0.5 fiber
"Healthified" Recipe: 195 calories, 3 carbs, 1.5 fiber

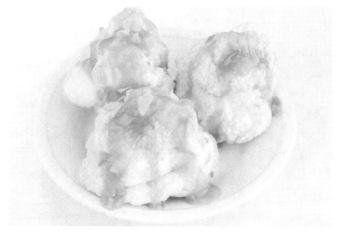

Cupcakes:
3 eggs, separated
1/4 cup Erythritol and 1 tsp Stevia Glycerite
4 TBS melted butter or coconut oil
1/2 cup of blanched almond flour
1/4 Celtic sea salt
1/4 tsp baking soda
1 tsp vanilla
1/4 tsp cinnamon (optional)
2 TBS cocoa powder
Frosting:
1 ChocoPerfection Bar
1 TBS unsweetened almond milk (or cream)

Whip the egg whites until stiff peaks form. Combine the yolks, sweetener, oil/butter and whisk until well-blended. Combine all the dry ingredients, blend well. Gently fold the wet ingredients into the whipped whites and then slowly fold in the dry mixture, add vanilla and blend well. Fill the cupcake pan 3/4 of the way full. Bake for 15-18 minutes at 350 degrees F, or until a toothpick comes out clean. Meanwhile: Melt the chocolate bar (in 10 second intervals in microwave) and add in whipping cream. Once the donut is cooled, dip in melted ChocoPerfection Chocolate Bar!

Creamy Filling: Option 1 (lower calories, must be eaten the same day)
2 egg whites
2 drops of Stevia Glycerite

Whip egg whites to stiff peaks. Blend in sweetener and re-whip until stiff peaks form again. Place filling in filler tool (I used a ziplock and cut a tiny hole in the corner). Place cooled cupcake on its side and inject filling into it.

Creamy Filling: OPTION 2
1 cup heavy cream
2 drops of Stevia Glycerite

Whip the cream until light and fluffy, add in the sweetener. Use to fill cooled Little Debbie same as above.

Swirly White Topping:
Cream cheese

I placed cream cheese in a Ziploc bag. Cut a tiny corner out and swirled it out onto the chocolate. Makes 6 cupcakes.

Nutritional Information:
Using egg white filling: 195 calories, 5 carbs, 3.5 fiber, 1.5 net carbs
Using whipping cream filling: 297 calories, 6 carbs, 3.5 fiber, 2.5 net carbs

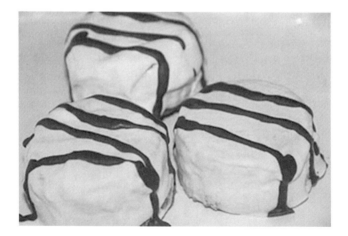

HOMEMADE HO-HOS

Cake:

4 eggs

1/2 cup Erythritol and 1 tsp Stevia Glycerite

5 TBS cocoa powder (preferably Dutch processed), plus more for dusting

2 tsp pure vanilla extract

1 cup blanched almond flour

1/4 cup Jay Robb vanilla/chocolate whey

1/4 tsp Celtic sea salt

5 TBS butter, melted

Water or Unsweetened Vanilla almond milk

Filling:

1/2 cup Erythritol and 1/2 tsp Stevia Glycerite

4 oz. cream cheese

1 1/2 cups heavy cream

1 tsp pure vanilla extract

Frosting:

2 cups ChocoPerfection Bar, chopped (or Simply Lite bars)

2 TBS unsweetened almond milk

Preheat oven to 350 degrees F. Butter a half sheet pan (17×12 inches), then line with parchment paper. Butter the paper and sides of pan and dust with cocoa powder. In a medium-sized, heat-proof bowl, set over a saucepan of simmering water; whisk together the eggs, sweetener, and 2 tablespoons of cocoa powder. Whisk almost constantly until mixture is warm to the touch. Remove from heat, and with an electric mixer, beat on high for several minutes until the mixture is smooth. Stir in vanilla. Combine the rest of the cocoa powder, almond flour, whey, and salt in small bowl. Fold in until well incorporated, followed by the melted butter. Spread evenly into prepared pan and bake for 10 minutes, or until cake springs back when touched. Remove the cake from the oven and let sit in the pan for 1 minute. Run a knife along the edge to release the cake then flip it out onto parchment paper. Brush the paper (the one you lined the pan with) with water or almond milk and let soak for 2 minutes. Peel it off the cake. Trim dry edges from the cake. Let cool covered with plastic wrap. While the cake cools, make the filling. In a medium-sized bowl, with an electric mixer, cream sweetener and cream cheese until smooth. In another bowl, whip the cream until stiff peaks form, then fold in the cream cheese mixture. Fold into vanilla. When the cake is fully cooled, cut into 12 equal pieces. Spread filling evenly over the cake, and take each section and carefully roll up, being careful not to break the cake. When all pieces are rolled up, place in the freezer to set for about 20 minutes. In a small, microwave safe bowl, combine the chocolate chips, and the almond milk. Microwave on high for 45 seconds. Stir, and microwave for 10 seconds more until all the chips are melted. Remove the ho-ho's from the freezer, cut off any filling oozing out the sides, and coat in the melted chocolate mixture. Place on parchment paper and return to the freezer until the frosting is set. Makes 12 servings.

NUTRITIONAL COMPARISON (per serving):
Hostess Ho Ho = 380 calories, 54 carbs, 1 fiber (53 effective carbs)
"Healthified" Ho Ho = 294 calories, 7.5 carbs, 4.1 fiber (3.4 effective carbs)

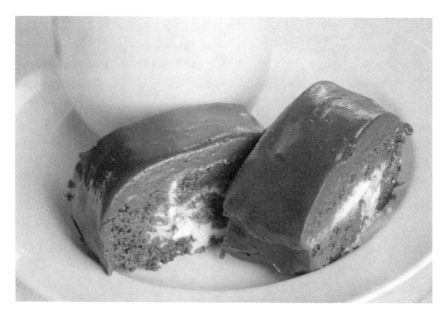

TWINKIES

1/4 cup coconut flour
1/4 tsp Celtic sea salt
1/2 tsp baking soda
3 eggs
1/3 cup Erythritol and 1/2 tsp Stevia Glycerite
1/2 TBS vanilla
1/4 cup butter or coconut oil
CHOCOLATE OPTION: add 3 TBS cocoa powder

Preheat oven to 350 degrees F. Blend all the dry ingredients and then start adding all the wet ingredients to the dry mix. Blend the mixture well. Pour the batter into the boats (or cupcake liners) and fill 3/4 of the way. Bake for about 12 minutes, or until a toothpick comes out clean. Cool the cakes. Fill the Twinkie using a decorator tool that came with the pan, or a pastry bag.

Creamy Filling: Option 1 (lighter in calories)
2 egg whites
2 drops of Stevia Glycerite

Whip egg whites to stiff peaks. Blend in sweetener and re-whip until stiff peaks form again. Place filling in Twinkie filling injector. Place cooled Twinkie flat side up and inject filling into Twinkie in 3 spots on its flat (bottom) side.

Creamy Filling: OPTION 2
1/2 cup heavy cream
2 to 3 drops of Stevia Glycerite)

Whip the cream until light and fluffy, add in the sweetener. Use to fill cooled Twinkie.

Nutritional Information (per Twinkie)
Using egg white filling = 199 calories, 4.75 carbs, 2 fiber

Using whipping cream filling = 297 calories, 6 carbs, 2.5 fiber

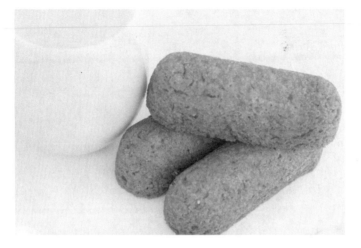

45 CALORIE CHOCOLATE PUDDING

3/4 cup chocolate unsweetened almond milk
1/2 tsp guar gum or Xanthan
1 TBS cocoa powder
Stevia Glycerite to taste

Place in a medium sized bowl and blend until smooth. Let sit for 5 minutes to "set." The mixture will thicken up. Enjoy!

NUTRITIONAL COMPARISON:
JELL-O Fat-Free chocolate pudding = 93 calories, 21 carbs, 0.3 fiber
Almond milk pudding = 45 calories, 5 carbs, 2.7g fiber

PEANUT BUTTER CUP CUPCAKES

2 cups peanut flour
1/2 cup Erythritol and 1/2 tsp Stevia Glycerite
3 1/2 tsp aluminum free baking powder
1 tsp Celtic sea salt
1/8 tsp baking soda
3 tsp baking cocoa
1 1/4 cups vanilla or chocolate almond milk
1 tsp vanilla
3 large eggs

Preheat oven to 350 degrees F. Line cupcake pans with paper liners or you may also grease cupcake pans with butter. Combine all ingredients in a large mixing bowl. Mix at low speed for 30 seconds while scraping bowl. Mix at high speed for 3 minutes, scraping bowl every minute. Spoon cupcake batter into liners until they are 2/3 full. You should have enough batter for 24 cupcakes. Bake for 20 to 25 minutes or until toothpick inserted in center comes out clean. Cool 10 minutes in pans then move to wire rack to cool completely. Frost cupcakes any way you want. Try just spreading extra peanut butter as your frosting.

Peanut Flour (Per CUP): 196 calories, 20.82 carbs, 9.5g fiber, 31.3g protein

Makes 6 LARGE cupcakes (per cupcake): 110 calories, 7.6 carbs, 3g fiber, 14g protein!

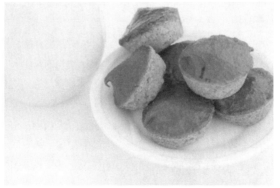

COCONUT STRAWBERRY POPS

1 cup coconut milk (I used Trader Joe's)
1 cup sliced strawberries
2 to 3 drops Stevia Glycerite

Mix the coconut milk and sweetener together. Slowly add the strawberries (they will probably make the milk red). Place in Popsicle molds and freeze. Serves 4.

Nutritional Information (per serving) = 49 calories, 4.4 carbs, .7 fiber

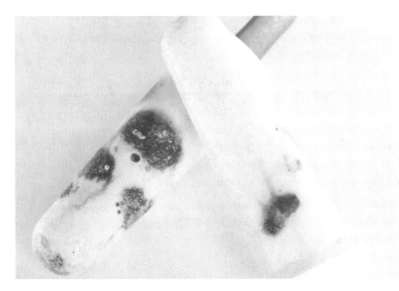

FUDGE-CICLES

2 oz. cream cheese
1 cup chocolate (or vanilla) unsweetened almond milk
4 drops Stevia Glycerite
3 TBS unsweetened cocoa powder

Mix all together and place in popsicle makers. Makes 4 servings.

Nutritional Information (per serving) = 80 calories, 4 carbs, 1.2 fiber

ICE CREAM SANDWICHES

1/2 cup vanilla whey protein
3/4 cup almond flour
1/4 tsp baking soda
4 TBS cocoa powder
1/4 tsp Celtic sea salt
1/4 cup butter
1/4 tsp Stevia Glycerite
2 TBS water (to hold dough together)

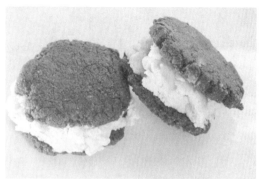

Ice Cream Filling:
2 oz. heavy cream
2 oz. cream cheese
3 TBS Natural creamy peanut butter (OR more cream cheese)
2-4 TBS erythritol and 1/2 tsp Stevia Glycerite

Preheat the oven to 350 degrees F. In a medium bowl, stir together the whey, almond flour, cocoa, baking soda and salt. Cut in the butter using a pastry blender or your fingers until the butter lumps are smaller than peas. Stir in the water and sweetener to form a stiff dough. On a cookie sheet, place 1/4 inch thick rectangles 2 inches apart. I used my hands to shape into rectangles (about 2 inches wide, by 4 inches long). Bake for 12-14 minutes in the preheated oven, until edges are lightly browned. Cool in oven to crisp up. ICE CREAM FILLING: In a medium sized bowl, mix heavy cream with a mixer until it forms stiff peaks. Do not over-beat or it will turn into butter! Set the cream aside. Beat cream cheese, sweetener, and peanut butter until the mixture is smooth and clump free. Test for sweetness. It should be a bit sweeter than you want the finished product. Using a spatula, gently fold cream cheese into the whipped cream. Freeze for 1/2 hour. Once it has hardened enough to handle, remove from freezer and fill in between 2 "cookies." Place back in freezer to set.

NUTRITIONAL Comparison:
Store Bought = 200 calories, 41 carbs, trace fiber
"Healthified" = 150 calories, 5 carbs, 2 fiber

STRAWBERRY CHEESECAKE POPS

I LOVE Ben and Jerry's Strawberry Cheesecake Ice cream. But check out these stats! 230 calories, 13g Fat, 27g carbs, 21g sugar, 3 protein

Eat this instead:

1 cup strawberries, sliced

4 oz. cream cheese, softened

1/4 cup unsweetened vanilla almond milk

8 drops Stevia Glycerite (or more to taste)*

*Could also use 4 TBS Erythritol and 2 tsp Stevia Glycerite instead.

In a bowl, mix cream cheese, almond milk and sweetener until smooth. Slowly stir in slices of strawberries. Pour mixture into Popsicle molds. Place in freezer for at least 2 hours and serve. Serves 4.

Nutritional Information (per serving) = 125 calories, 4.8 carbs, 1.1g fiber

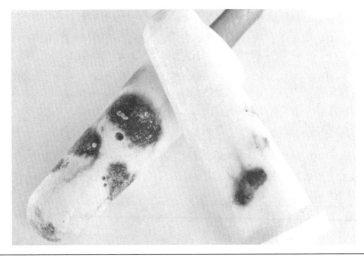

CHOCOLATE ZUCCHINI BROWNIES

1/2 cup coconut oil or butter, softened

3/4 cups Erythritol and 1 tsp Stevia Glycerite

2 tsp vanilla extract

2 cups peanut flour

1/2 cup unsweetened cocoa powder

1 1/2 tsp baking soda

1 tsp Celtic sea salt

2 cups shredded zucchini

1/2 cup chopped walnuts

(optional)

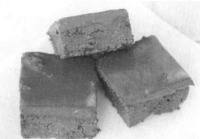

Frosting:

6 TBS unsweetened cocoa powder

1/4 cup butter

1/4 cup Erythritol (powdered)

1/4 cup vanilla almond milk

1/2 tsp vanilla extract

Preheat oven to 350 degrees F. Grease a 9x13 inch baking pan. In a large bowl, mix together the oil, sweetener and 2 teaspoons vanilla until well blended. Combine the peanut flour, 1/2 cup cocoa, baking soda and salt; stir into the sugar mixture. Fold in the zucchini and walnuts. NOTE: The batter will be crumbly, some of you might be tempted to add an egg, but don't. If you do, you will end up with a cake rather than a "fudgy" brownie. Spread evenly into the prepared pan. Bake for 25 to 30 minutes in the preheated oven, until brownies spring back when gently touched. To make the frosting, make Erythritol into a powder in a food processor. Melt together the 6 tablespoons of cocoa and butter; set aside to cool. In a medium bowl, blend together the sweetener, almond milk and 1/2 teaspoon vanilla. Stir in the cocoa mixture. Spread over cooled brownies before cutting into squares. Makes 16 servings.

Nutritional Information (per serving) = 117 calories, 5.7 carbs, 2.9g fiber, 6g protein

FLOUR-LESS CHOCOLATE TIRAMISU TORTE

Chocolate Torte:

7 oz. unsweetened chocolate

1 3/4 sticks salted butter

1 1/4 cup Erythritol

2 TBS Stevia Glycerite

5 large eggs

Mascarpone filling:

1 8-oz. package mascarpone (or cream cheese)

1 tsp Stevia Glycerite (to taste)

1 egg

Preheat oven to 375 degrees F. Grease a muffin tin. Set aside. Brown the butter (if desired…tastes way better!) in a saucepan. Once the butter is brown (not black!), slowly add the chocolate. Add the sweetener. Let cool in fridge. Once cool, add one egg at a time using a mixer. Cream filling: Mix mascarpone cheese, sweetener and egg. Fill the muffin tins with chocolate filling and a dollop of cheese in the middle. Bake for 25 minutes. I inverted my torte; I thought it looked better that way. Enjoy! Serves 16.

Nutritional Information (per serving) = 212 calories, 4.1 carbs, 2 fiber

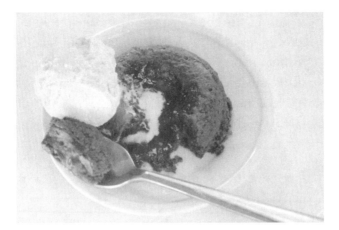

FLOUR-LESS CHOCOLATE TORTE

7 oz unsweetened chocolate
1 3/4 sticks salted butter
1 1/4 cup erythritol
2 TBS Stevia Glycerite
5 large eggs
1 TBS peanut flour (optional)

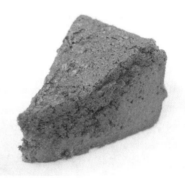

Preheat oven to 375 degrees F.
Grease an 8 inch pan and line
with parchment paper
(greased or mini muffin tins). Grease parchment paper. Brown the butter
(if desired…tastes way better!) in a saucepan. Once the butter is brown
(not black!), slowly add the chocolate (don't burn the chocolate). Add the
sweetener. Let cool in fridge. Once cool, add one egg at a time. Last add
the peanut flour. Bake for 25 minutes. Serve with cream cheese frosting.

<u>Cream Cheese frosting</u>:
1 stick salted butter
8 oz. cream cheese
3 TBS Vanilla Almond Milk
1 TBS Stevia Glycerite (to taste)

Brown the butter in a sauce pan (stir constantly on high heat until light
golden brown – it makes such a difference!!!). Once brown add the cream
cheese, almond milk, and sweetener to taste. Mix until creamy and allow
it to cool for at least 2 hours, it will thicken. Spread on top of cake (add
almonds if desired) and enjoy. Makes 16 servings.

Nutritional Information (per serving) = 285 Calories, 5 carbs, 2.3g fiber,
5g protein

CHOCOLATE LAVA CAKES

6 oz. dark chocolate ChocoPerfection Bar
1/4 cup vanilla almond milk
1 stick unsalted butter
2 eggs
2 egg yolks
1/3 cup Erythritol
1/2 tsp Stevia Glycerite
1/2 tsp vanilla extract
1/4 cup peanut flour

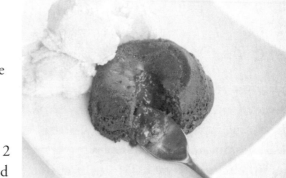

To make centers, melt 2 ounces of chocolate and vanilla almond milk in double boiler. Whisk gently to blend. Refrigerate about 2 hours or until firm. Form into 6 balls; refrigerate until needed. To make cake, heat oven to 400 degrees F. Spray six 4-ounce ramekins or custard cups with cooking spray. Melt 4 ounces of chocolate and butter in double boiler; whisk gently to blend. With an electric mixer, whisk eggs, yolks, sweetener, and vanilla on high speed about 5 minutes or until thick and light. Fold melted chocolate mixture and peanut flour into egg mixture just until combined. Spoon cake batter into ramekins. Place a chocolate ball in the middle of each ramekin. Bake about 15 minutes or until cake is firm to the touch. Let it sit out of the oven for about 5 minutes. Run a small, sharp knife around inside of each ramekin, place a plate on top, invert and remove ramekin. Garnish with a dollop of whipped cream. Serves 6.

NUTRITIONAL COMPARISON:
"Traditional Lava Cake" = 424 calories, 31.8 carbs, 0.2 fiber, 4.9 protein
"Healthified" Lava Cakes: 290 calories, 9.3 carbs, 7.6 fiber, 6.9 protein

PECAN SPICE CAKE WITH CREAM CHEESE FROSTING

2 3/4 cups blanched almond flour

2 tsp baking powder

1 tsp baking soda

3/4 tsp Celtic sea salt

1 TBS ground cinnamon

1 1/4 tsp freshly grated nutmeg

1 tsp ground ginger

1/2 tsp ground allspice

1/4 tsp ground cloves

1 1/2 sticks unsalted butter, cut into 1-inch pieces and softened

1 1/2 cups Erythritol and 1.5 tsp Stevia Glycerite

3 large eggs at room temperature 30 minutes

1 1/2 tsp pure vanilla extract

1 1/2 cups sour cream

3/4 cup pecans, toasted and finely chopped

For frosting:

3 (8-oz.) packages cream cheese, softened

1 1/2 sticks unsalted butter, softened

2-3 TBS vanilla almond milk

1 tsp Stevia Glycerite (to taste)

1 1/3 cups pecans, toasted and finely chopped (optional for outside)

Make cake: Preheat oven to 350 degrees F. Grease cake pans. Sift together almond flour, baking powder, baking soda, salt, and spices into a large bowl. In another bowl, beat together butter (1 1/2 sticks) and sweetener with an electric mixer at medium-high speed until pale and fluffy, 3 to 5 minutes. Beat in eggs 1 at a time, beating well after each addition, then beat in vanilla. Reduce speed to low, add flour mixture and sour cream alternately in batches, beginning and ending with flour mixture and mixing until batter is just smooth. Mix in pecans until just combined. Spoon batter evenly into pans, smoothing tops, then rap pans once or twice to expel any air bubbles. Bake until pale golden and a wooden pick inserted in center of cakes comes out clean, 30 to 35 minutes. Cool 10 minutes in pans on racks. Run a thin knife around edge of pans, then invert racks over pans and re-invert cakes onto racks to cool completely.

<u>Make frosting</u>: Beat together cream cheese, butter, and almond milk in a bowl with clean beaters at medium-high speed until fluffy, 1 to 2 minutes. Sift in sweetener and beat at medium-high speed until frosting is smooth.

Assemble and frost cake: Halve each cake layer horizontally with a long serrated knife using a gentle sawing motion. Put 1 layer, cut side up, on a cake stand or large plate and spread with about 3/4 cup frosting. Stack remaining cake layers, spreading about 3/4 cup frosting on each layer and ending with top cake layer cut side down. Spread top and side of cake with remaining frosting (about 3 1/2 cups) and coat side of cake with pecans (1 1/3 cups), gently pressing to help them adhere. Serves 18.

Nutritional Information (per slice) = 422 calories, 6.5 carbs, 2.1 fiber

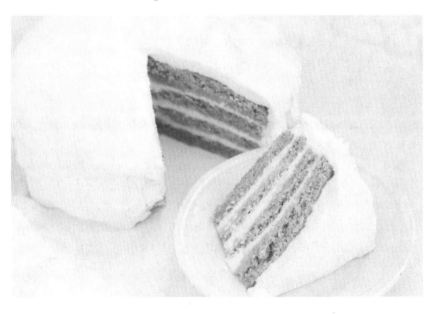

CANNOLI

Shell:

1 egg white

1 TBS butter (melted)

1 oz. cream cheese
(softened)

1/4 cup almond flour

1/4 cup vanilla whey
protein

Filling:

3/4 cup whole milk ricotta
cheese (drained w/ cheesecloth & squeezed dry)

3/4 cup mascarpone cheese (or cream cheese)

1 tsp Stevia Glycerite (to taste)

1/2 tsp vanilla

1/2 tsp ground cinnamon

A pinch of salt

Heat a pizzelle skillet on high. Whip the white until frothy, not stiff. Add the almond flour, vanilla whey and other ingredients. Mix until smooth. Place 1 TBS dough onto greased skillet, close tightly. Let sit for 1-3 minutes depending on skillet directions. While you are removing, before it cools, roll into a cylinder shape. Set aside to cool. To make filling: Mix filling ingredients together. Cover and refrigerate until ready to use. Use a Ziploc (cut the corner) and pipe into the shells. Let the filling smoosh out of each end of the shells. Keep refrigerated until serving. Makes 14 servings.

NUTRITIONAL COMPARISON (per cannoli):
Traditional Cannoli: 250 calories, 44 carbs, trace fiber
"Healthified" Cannoli = 97 calories, 1.6 carbs, trace fiber

CREME BRULEE

6 egg yolks
6 TBS Erythritol and 1 drop Stevia Glycerite
1/2 tsp vanilla extract (I used 1 vanilla bean)
2 1/2 cups heavy cream

Preheat oven to 300 degrees F. Beat egg yolks, 4 tablespoons Erythritol, stevia and vanilla in a mixing bowl until thick and creamy. Pour cream and vanilla bean (if using) into a saucepan and stir over low heat until it almost comes to boil. Remove the cream from heat immediately. Stir cream into the egg yolk mixture; beat until combined. Pour cream mixture into the top of a double boiler. Stir over simmering water until mixture lightly coats the back of a spoon; approximately 3 minutes. Remove mixture from heat immediately and pour into a shallow heat-proof dish. Bake in preheated oven for 30 minutes. Remove from oven and cool to room temperature. Refrigerate for 1 hour, or overnight.

Preheat oven to broil. Sift the remaining sweetener evenly over custard. Place dish under broiler until sweetener melts, about 2 minutes. Watch carefully so as not to burn. Remove from heat and allow it to cool. Refrigerate until custard is set again. Makes 6 servings.

Nutritional Information (per serving) = 368 calories, 3.1g carbs, trace fiber, 2.3g protein

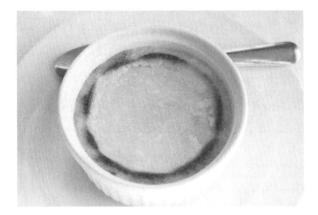

VANILLA BEAN CHEESECAKE

Crust:
2 cups Macadamia nuts,
ground fine
4 TBS Erythritol
1/4 tsp Stevia Glycerite
4 TBS Butter
Filling:
6 (8 oz.) packages cream
cheese
3 eggs
3/4 cup Erythritol
1 vanilla bean

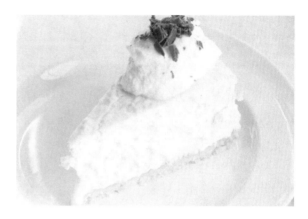

Preheat oven to 350 degrees F. Mix the "crust" ingredients and then press into bottom of spring-form pan. Cut a vanilla bean open through the middle and scrape the beans out of the inside with a sharp knife. Optional: in a coffee grinder, blend Erythritol until a fine powder. This creates a smoother cheesecake. Mix cream cheese, sweetener, vanilla bean with an electric mixer until blended. Add eggs one at a time, mixing on low after each, just until blended. Pour over crust. I use a water bath to create a more even baking process. To prevent water from seeping into the removable bottom of the spring form pan, wrap aluminum foil completely around the bottom and halfway up the sides of the pan. Place the cheesecake into a jellyroll pan (or any baking pan with sides) and place the pans into the oven. Use a teakettle to fill the outer pan with hot water. Bake 1 hour and 5 minutes to 1 hour and 10 minutes or until center is almost set. Run knife around the rim of the pan to loosen cake and allow it to cool before removing the spring-form pan ring. Refrigerate overnight. Serves 18.

NUTRITIONAL COMPARISON:
Cheesecake Factory Vanilla Bean: 869 calories, 72 carbs, 1 fiber, 3 protein
"Healthified" Cheesecake = 407 calories, 4.8 carbs, 1.2 fiber, 3 protein

PUMPKIN SWIRL CHEESECAKE

CRUST:
1 cup almond flour
1 cup finely chopped pecans
1/4 cup butter or coconut oil,
melted
4 TBS Erythritol and 1/2
tsp Stevia Glycerite
FILLING:
3 8-oz pkgs Cream Cheese,
softened
3/4 cup Erythritol, divided
1 tsp vanilla
3 eggs
1 cup canned pumpkin
1 tsp ground cinnamon
1/4 tsp ground nutmeg
1 dash ground cloves

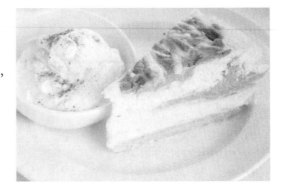

Heat oven to 350 degrees F. CRUST: Combine almond flour, pecans, Erythritol, stevia and butter. Press onto bottom of 9 inch spring form pan. FILLING: Beat cream cheese, 1/2 cup of the erythritol and vanilla with electric mixer until well blended. Add eggs, one at a time, mixing on low speed after each addition just until blended. Remove 1 cup plain batter; place in small bowl. Stir remaining 1/4 cup erythritol, pumpkin and spices into remaining batter. Spoon pumpkin batter into crust; top with spoonfuls of reserved plain batter. Cut through batters with knife several times for marble effect. Bake 45 minutes or until center is almost set. Cool completely. Refrigerate 4 hours or overnight. Cut into 12 slices. Store leftover cheesecake in refrigerator.
Serves 12

NUTRITIONAL COMPARISON:
Traditional Cheesecake = 375 calories, 30.4 carbs, 1 fiber
"Healthified" Cheesecake = 333 calories, 3.7 carbs, 1.5 fiber

PEANUT BUTTER CUP CHEESECAKE

Crust:
1/4 cup Erythritol and 1/2 tsp Stevia Glycerite
3/4 cup vanilla whey (Jay Robb)
3/4 cup peanut flour
1/2 cup butter, softened
1/2 tsp Celtic sea salt

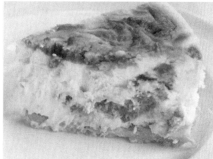

Filling:
6 (8 oz.) packages cream cheese
3 eggs
3/4 cup Erythritol
1 tsp vanilla extract (or 1 vanilla bean)

Peanut Butter Swirl:
1 cup natural peanut butter
1/8 cup Erythritol and 1/4 tsp Stevia Glycerite
1/4 cup almond milk (or cream)
ChocoPerfection Chips

Preheat oven to 350 degrees F. Mix the "crust" ingredients and then press into bottom of spring-form pan. If using vanilla bean: Cut a vanilla bean open through the middle and scrape the beans out of the inside with a sharp knife. Option: in a coffee grinder, blend erythritol until a fine powder. This creates a smoother cheesecake. Mix the peanut butter swirl ingredients together until smooth and set aside. Mix cream cheese, sweetener, vanilla with an electric mixer until blended. Add eggs one at a time, mixing on low after each, just until blended. Pour over crust. Then using a knife swirl in the peanut butter mix. I use a water bath to create a more even baking process. To prevent water from seeping into the removable bottom of the spring form pan, wrap aluminum foil completely around the bottom and halfway up the sides of the pan. Place the cheesecake into a jellyroll pan (or any baking pan with sides) and place the pans into the oven. Use a teakettle to fill the outer pan with hot water. Bake 1 hour and 5 minutes to 1 hour and 10 minutes or until

center is almost set. Run knife around the rim of the pan to loosen cake and allow it to cool before removing the spring-form pan ring. If desired push chocolate chips into the side of the cheesecake. Refrigerate overnight. NOTE: I melted a ChocoPerfection Bar with 4 TBS vanilla almond milk and swirled it into the top instead. Serves 18.
NUTRITIONAL COMPARISON:
Cheesecake Factory Cheesecake = 930 calories, 93 carbs, 1 fiber
"HEALTHIFIED" Cheesecake = 407 calories, 4.8 carbs, 1.2 fiber, 3 protein

ICE CREAM CONE

1 egg white
1 TBS butter (melted)
1 oz. cream cheese (softened)
1/4 cup almond flour
1/4 cup vanilla whey protein

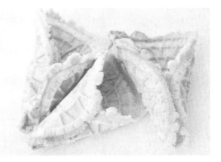

Heat a pizzelle skillet on high. Whip the white until frothy, not stiff. Add the almond flour, vanilla whey and other ingredients. Mix until smooth. Place 1 tablespoon dough onto greased skillet, close tightly. Let sit for 1-3 minutes depending on skillet directions. While you are removing, before it cools, roll into a cone shape. Makes 14 cones.

NUTRITIONAL COMPARISON (per cone)
Traditional Sugar CONE = 114 calories, 23.8 carbs, 0.5 fiber
"Healthified" Sugar Cone = 35 calories, 0.5 carbs, trace fiber

BOSTON CREAM CHEESECAKE

<u>For cake:</u>
1 1/2 cups blanched almond flour
1 tsp baking powder
1/2 tsp baking soda
1/2 tsp Celtic sea salt
3/4 stick butter, cut into 1-inch pieces and softened
3/4 cups erythritol and 1 tsp Stevia Glycerite
3 large eggs
1 tsp pure vanilla extract
3/4 cups sour cream
<u>Filling:</u>
3 (8 oz.) packages cream cheese, softened
1/4 cup, plus 2 TBS Erythritol and 1 tsp Stevia Glycerite
2 tsp. vanilla extract, divided
3 large eggs
3/4 cup sour cream
2 oz. unsweetened baking chocolate
3 TBS unsweetened vanilla almond milk
2 TBS unsalted butter or coconut oil
1 tsp Stevia Glycerite (or sweetener to taste)

<u>Make cake:</u> Put oven rack in middle position and preheat oven to 350 degrees F. Grease a cake pan. Sift together almond flour, baking powder, baking soda, and salt into a large bowl. In another bowl, beat together butter and sweetener with an electric mixer at medium-high speed until pale and fluffy, 3 to 5 minutes. Beat in eggs 1 at a time, beating well after each addition, then beat in vanilla. Reduce speed to low, then add flour mixture and sour cream alternately in batches, beginning and ending with flour mixture and mixing until batter is just smooth. Spoon batter into pan, smoothing top. Bake until pale golden and a wooden pick inserted in center of cake comes out clean, 30-35 minutes. Cool 10 minutes in pan on racks. Run a thin knife around edge of pan, then invert rack over pan and reinvert cake onto rack to cool completely.
<u>Cheesecake Layer:</u> Beat cream cheese, sweetener and 1 tsp of the vanilla

with electric mixer on medium speed until well blended. Add eggs, 1 at a time, mixing on low speed after each addition just until blended. Blend in sour cream; pour over cake layer. Bake at 325 degrees F for 40 to 45 minutes or until center is almost set if using a silver spring form pan. (Bake at 300 degrees F for 40 to 45 minutes or until center is almost set if using a dark nonstick spring form pan.) Run knife or metal spatula around rim of pan to loosen cake; cool before removing rim of pan. Topping: Place chocolate, milk and butter in medium bowl. Melt chocolate in a double boiler or microwave on HIGH 2 minutes or until butter is melted, stirring after 1 minute. Stir until chocolate is completely melted (don't burn the chocolate!). Add sweetener and remaining 1 tsp. vanilla; mix well. Spread over cooled cheesecake. Refrigerate 4 hours or overnight. Makes 12 servings.

NUTRITIONAL COMPARISON (per serving)
Traditional Boston Cheesecake = 563 calories, 59 carbs, 1.1 fiber
"Healthified" Boston Cheesecake = 461 calories, 8 carbs, 2.2 fiber

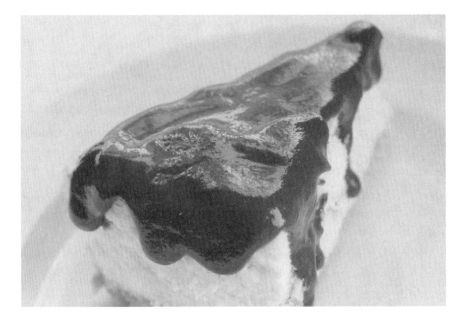

PUMPKIN PIE

1/2 cup vanilla whey or egg white protein
3/4 cup almond flour
1/4 tsp Celtic sea salt
1/4 cup butter or coconut oil
4 drops Stevia Glycerite
1-2 TBS water (just enough to hold dough together)
FILLING:
1 (15 oz.) can pumpkin
1 cup Coconut Milk (OR cream cheese)
1 tsp pure vanilla or maple extract
1/2 tsp ground cinnamon
1/2 tsp Celtic sea salt
1/4 tsp ginger
1/4 tsp nutmeg
3/4 cup Erythritol and 1/2 tsp Stevia Glycerite
3 TBS gelatin
1/4 cup hot water

Preheat oven to 350 degrees F. CRUST: In a large bowl cream the butter and sweetener together until very smooth. Sift the salt and whey into the almond flour, then slowly add the almond flour mixture into the butter mixture. Mix until well combined, then slowly add water just until the dough is soft, yet able to roll out. Form into a tight ball and cool in the fridge to chill. place into an 8 by 8 pie pan and spread out over the bottom. FILLING: In large mixing bowl, dissolve gelatin in 1/4 cup boiling water. Combine pumpkin, coconut milk, cinnamon, maple flavoring, ginger, nutmeg, sweetener and salt; mix into the gelatin. Pour into pie shell. Cover the edges of the pie with aluminum foil (otherwise it will burn). Bake at 350 degrees F for 70 minutes or until set in the middle. Top with whipped cream or coconut cream and enjoy! Store covered in refrigerator.
NUTRITIONAL COMPARISON (per slice, serves 8):
Using traditional Evaporated Milk: 379 calories, 30.5 carbs, 3 fiber
Using Coconut Milk: 210 calories, 7.1 carbs, 3 fiber

BÛCHE DE NOËL

Filling:
2 cups heavy cream
4 TBS Erythritol and 1/4 tsp Stevia Glycerite
1/2 cup unsweetened cocoa powder (optional)
1 tsp vanilla extract
Cake:
6 eggs, separated
6 TBS Erythritol
1/3 cup unsweetened cocoa powder
1 1/2 tsp vanilla extract
1/8 tsp Celtic sea salt

Preheat oven to 375 degrees F. Line a 10x15 inch jellyroll pan with parchment paper. In a large bowl, whip cream, 4 TBS erythritol, 1/2 cup cocoa (if using), and 1 teaspoon vanilla until thick and stiff. Refrigerate. In a large bowl, use an electric mixer to beat egg yolks with 6 TBS erythritol until thick and pale. Blend in 1/3 cup cocoa, 1 1/2 teaspoons vanilla, and salt. In large dry bowl, using clean beaters, whip egg whites until stiff peaks. Immediately fold the yolk mixture into the whites. Spread the batter evenly into the prepared pan. Bake for 12 to 15 minutes in the preheated oven, or until the cake springs back when lightly touched. Run a knife around the edge of the pan, and turn the warm cake out onto a clean dishtowel. Remove and discard parchment paper. Starting at the short edge of the cake, roll the cake up with the towel. Cool for 30 minutes. Unroll the cake, and spread the filling to within 1 inch of the edge. Roll the cake up with the filling inside. Place seam side down onto a serving plate, and refrigerate until serving. Dust with cocoa powder and melted ChocoPerfection bar or frost with homemade "healthified" chocolate frosting (found in previous recipe) before serving. Serves 12.

NUTRITIONAL COMPARISON (compared without frosting added)
Traditional Buche de Noel = 279 calories, 27.4 carbs, 2 fiber, 5 protein
"Healthified" Buche de Noel = 209 calories, 2.8 carbs, 0.8 fiber

ANGEL FOOD CAKE

1 cup vanilla whey protein
2 tsp baking powder
1/8 tsp Celtic sea salt
1/2 tsp cream of tartar
5 large eggs, separated
7 TBS Erythritol and 1 tsp Stevia Glycerite
2 tsp vanilla extract
3/4 cup unsweetened vanilla almond milk
Glaze:
2 oz heavy cream (or Unsweetened vanilla almond milk)
2 TBS butter
1 tsp vanilla extract or lemon extract
3 oz cream cheese
Sweetener to taste (if desired)

Preheat oven to 300 degrees F. Spray a Bundt pan with olive oil spray very well. Sift protein powder, baking powder, and salt and set aside. In a large bowl, beat egg whites with cream of tartar until stiff. In another bowl, beat egg yolks, sweetener, and vanilla. Beat in almond milk, and then beat in dry ingredients. Fold into whites very carefully, and then spoon into a prepared Bundt pan. Bake for 45 minutes, then let cool 10 minutes before inverting and removing (this is the tricky part, just do your best). For the glaze, beat the cream, butter, cream cheese and vanilla (sweetener if desired) well. If this is too thick, add more cream, 1 tablespoon at a time. Drizzle over cooled cake. Makes 12 servings.

Nutritional Info (per serving): 114 Calories, 9g Fat, 13g Protein, 1carb, trace Fiber

"RICE" PUDDING

1/2 cup finely grated (riced) RAW cauliflower
1/2 cup coconut milk (or Heavy Cream)
2 or 3 drops Stevia Glycerite (to taste)
1 tsp vanilla extract
1/2 tsp cinnamon
2 egg yolks
1/2 cup unsweetened almond milk
4 oz cream cheese

Prepare the cauliflower by placing it in a food processor and pulsing until small, rice-like pieces. Place in a microwave-safe bowl and add 1/4 cup coconut milk with sweetener, extracts, cinnamon. Heat in microwave for 1 1/2 minutes. Let stand for 15 minutes. Beat egg yolks 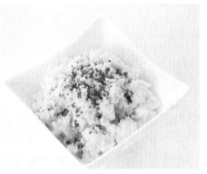 with 1/4 cup of coconut milk; set aside. Pour remainder of coconut milk and almond milk in sauce pan, add cream cheese and cook on medium heat, stirring constantly, until thickened. Add cauliflower mixture and egg mixture to pan and stir to re-thicken. Pour into 4 small ramekins or pudding dishes and refrigerate 1-3 hours. Serve and enjoy! Makes 4 servings.

NUTRITIONAL COMPARISON (per serving):
STORE Brand = 179 calories, 33 carbs, 1 fiber
"Healthified" Pudding = 155 calories, 1.5 carbs, trace fiber

EXTREME CHOCOLATE BIRTHDAY CAKE

1 1/4 cup Erythritol and 1 tsp Stevia Glycerite

1 3/4 cups peanut flour

3/4 cup unsweetened cocoa powder

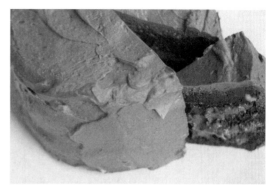

1 1/2 tsp baking soda

1 1/2 tsp baking powder

1 tsp Celtic sea salt

2 eggs

1 cup unsweetened vanilla almond milk

1/2 cup coconut oil or butter

2 tsp vanilla extract

1 cup boiling water

Frosting:

3/4 cup butter

3 oz. cream cheese

1 1/2 cups unsweetened cocoa powder

2 cups Erythritol (ground in coffee grinder into a powder)

3/4 cup unsweetened vanilla almond milk

1 tsp vanilla extract

Preheat oven to 350 degrees F. Grease two 9 inch cake pans. In a medium bowl, stir together the sweetener, peanut flour, cocoa, baking soda, baking powder and salt. Add the eggs, almond milk, oil and vanilla, mix for 3 minutes with an electric mixer. Stir in the boiling water by hand. Pour evenly into the two prepared pans. Bake for 30 to 35 minutes in the preheated oven, until a toothpick inserted comes out clean. Cool for 10 minutes before removing from pans to cool completely.

To make the frosting, use the second set of ingredients. Cream butter and cream cheese until light and fluffy. Stir in the cocoa and erythritol (powdered) alternately with the milk and vanilla. Beat to a spreading consistency. Split the layers of cooled cake horizontally, cover the top of each layer with frosting, then stack them onto a serving plate. Frost the outside of the cake. Serves 12.

NUTRITIONAL COMPARISON (per serving):

Using white flour, skim milk and sugar = 655 calories, 111 carbs, 5.8 fiber

Using peanut flour, almond milk = 314 calories, 13.8 carbs, 7.1 fiber

FLOATING ISLANDS

2 egg whites
1 pinch Celtic sea salt
3 TBS erythritol 3 drops Stevia Glycerite
3 cups unsweetened vanilla almond milk
3 eggs
2 egg yolks
1/4 cup Erythritol and 1/2 tsp Stevia Glycerite
1 1/2 tsp vanilla extract

In a medium bowl, beat egg whites with salt until foamy. Gradually pour in sweetener, beating until stiff peaks form. Bring almond milk to a simmer in large saucepan over medium heat. Drop egg white mixture in six separate mounds into simmering almond milk, leaving one inch between mounds. Poach 3 to 5 minutes, turning once. Remove meringues with slotted spoon and drain. Remove milk from heat and set aside. Beat eggs and egg yolks in a large bowl. Beat in 1/4 cup Erythritol and stevia. Stir in almond milk from the saucepan. Cook milk mixture in a double boiler over simmering water, stirring constantly, until mixture thickens enough to coat the back of a metal spoon. Let cool before stirring in vanilla. To serve, pour custard in a dish and top with poached meringues. Makes 4 servings.

Nutritional Information (per serving) = 118 calories, 2g carbs, 1 fiber, 12g protein

GERMAN CHOCOLATE CAKE

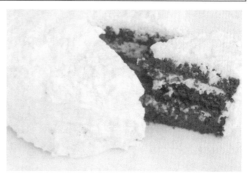

<u>Cake:</u>
2/3 cup butter or coconut oil
1 cup unsweetened cocoa powder
8 egg whites
1/4 tsp cream of tartar
1 cup coconut milk
2 whole eggs
8 egg yolks
1 cup Erythritol and 2 tsp Stevia Glycerite
1 tsp Celtic sea salt
1 tsp vanilla (or coconut extract)
1 cup coconut flour

In a saucepan, melt the coconut oil (or butter) over medium heat. Add cocoa powder and mix well. Remove from heat and cool. In a separate bowl, beat egg whites and cream of tartar until stiff peaks form; set aside. In another bowl mix together coconut milk, 2 whole eggs, 8 egg yolks, sweetener, salt, and vanilla. Slowly mix in cocoa mixture. Add coconut flour into batter and mix until it is very smooth. Fold egg whites into batter. Pour batter into 2 greased round 8 or 9x11/2-inch layer cake pans. Bake at 350 degrees F for 30-35 minutes or until a toothpick inserted into the center comes out clean. Cool (I put mine in the freezer overnight...it frosts really easy then). Fill layers and cover top and sides of cake with Coconut-Pecan Frosting.

<u>Coconut Frosting:</u>
1/4 cup coconut milk
8 oz. cream cheese
1/2 cup Erythritol and 1/2 tsp Stevia Glycerite
1/2 cup coconut oil or butter
1 tsp coconut extract
1 cup flaked coconut
1/2 cup pecans, chopped (or more to taste)

Mix coconut milk, cream cheese, sweetener, and butter until well combined and very smooth. Add extract, coconut, and pecans. Frost the cake and enjoy! Serves 16.

NUTRITIONAL COMPARISON:
Traditional German Chocolate Cake = 738 calories, 85.2 carbs, 1.8 fiber
"Healthified" German Chocolate Cake = 324 calories, 15 carbs, 9 fiber

RHUBARB BREAD PUDDING

2 cups eggplant, peeled
2 TBS butter or coconut oil, melted
1/2 cup Rhubarb, cut into 1/2 inch pieces
4 eggs, beaten
2 cups vanilla almond milk
1/4 cup Erythritol and 1/2
tsp Stevia Glycerite
1 tsp ground cinnamon
1 tsp vanilla extract

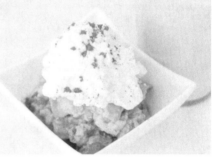

Preheat oven to 350 degrees F. Cut eggplant into 1 inch pieces and place in an 8 inch square baking pan. Drizzle melted butter over eggplant and add rhubarb. Bake for 15 minutes or until soft. In a medium mixing bowl, combine eggs, almond milk, sweetener, cinnamon, and vanilla. Beat until well mixed. Pour over eggplant, and lightly push down with a fork until eggplant is covered and soaking up the egg mixture. Bake in the preheated oven for 45 minutes, or until the top springs back when lightly tapped. Serve with a dollop of fresh whipped cream (sweetened with a drop of Stevia Glycerite). Makes 8 servings. For WHOLE BATCH = 616 calories, 20 carbs, 6 fiber

NUTRITIONAL COMPARISON (per serving):
Traditional Bread Pudding = 415 calories, 60 carbs, 0 fiber
Eggplant Bread Pudding = 77 calories, 2.5 carb, 0.8fiber

COCONUT CREAM PIE

Pie Crust:

1 egg white, whipped

4 drops Stevia Glycerite

1/4 cup coconut flour

2 TBS coconut oil or butter

2 TBS blanched almond flour

Preheat oven to 250 degrees F. Grease one 9 inch pie plate. In a small mixing bowl, beat egg whites until stiff peaks form. Beat in stevia. Fold in coconut, oil and almond flour. Press coconut mixture evenly along the bottom and sides of the pie plate. Bake for 10-14 minutes or golden color. Cool before filling with yummy goodness.

Filling:

2 cups (1 can) coconut milk

1/2 tsp Stevia Glycerite, plus 1/2 tsp for the egg whites

3 TBS coconut flour

3 eggs, separated

4 TBS cream cheese

1 tsp vanilla

1 3/4 cups unsweetened toasted coconut (optional for texture)

Preheat the oven to 400 degrees F. In a saucepan, whisk the coconut milk, stevia and coconut flour together. Place the pan over medium heat and bring the liquid up to a simmer. Remove from heat and add the cream cheese until smooth. Whisk the egg yolks together. Temper the hot coconut milk into the egg yolks. Whisk the egg mixture into the hot milk mixture. Bring the liquid up to a boil and reduce to a simmer. Cook the mixture, stirring constantly, until the filling is thick, about 4 to 6 minutes. Fold in the vanilla, and coconut (if using). Mix well. Pour the filling into the prepared pan and cool the pie completely. Using an electric mixer with a whip attachment, whip the egg white to soft peaks. Add the remaining sweetener and whip the egg white to stiff peaks. Spread the egg whites over the top of the pie. Place the pie in the oven for about 3 to 4 minutes, or until the meringue is golden brown.

BOSTON CREAM PIE

CAKE:

1/2 cup butter, melted

1/2 cup vanilla almond milk (or coconut milk)

9 eggs

1/2 cup Erythritol and 1/2 tsp Stevia Glycerite

3/4 tsp Celtic sea salt

1 tsp vanilla

3/4 cup sifted coconut flour

3/4 tsp baking powder

CREAM FILLING:

8 oz. cream cheese

4 TBS Butter

2 TBS unsweetened vanilla almond milk (or heavy cream)

2 TBS erythritol and 1/2 tsp Stevia Glycerite

Glaze:

4 oz. unsweetened chocolate, chopped

1 TBS butter, cut into four pieces

1/2 cup unsweetened almond milk (or heavy cream)

6 TBS Erythritol, powdered and 1/4 tsp Stevia Glycerite

To Make Cake: Preheat oven to 350 degrees F. Mix 1/2 cup butter, 1/2 cup almond milk, eggs, 1/2 cup sweetener, salt, and vanilla. Combine coconut flour with baking powder and whisk into batter until there are no lumps. Pour batter into greased 8x8x2-inch pan. Bake at 350 degrees F for 35 minutes or until knife inserted into center comes out clean. Cool. Once cooled, cut cake horizontally so you end up with 2 cakes. To make frosting: Mix all the ingredients together and fill in between the sheets of cake. To Make Glaze: Place 4 ounces chopped chocolate, 1 TBS butter, and 1/2 cup almond milk in a microwave safe bowl. Heat for 30 seconds, and stir until smooth. Mix in sweetener until smooth. Spread over assembled cake. Makes 16 servings.

Nutritional Information (per slice) = 229 Calories, 6.7 carbs, 3 fiber

CREAMY RHUBARB PIE

11/4 cup Erythritol plus 2 tsp Stevia Glycerite

1 8 oz. package cream cheese

2 eggs

2 TBS ground flaxseeds

1/2 tsp vanilla extract

1/4 tsp Celtic sea salt

3 cups chopped fresh rhubarb

1 (9 inch) unbaked pie shell (Recipe Follows)

PIE SHELL:

2 Cups Blanched almond flour

4 TBS Erythritol and 1/4 tsp Stevia Glycerite

4 TBS butter or coconut oil, melted

Topping:

1/3 cup Erythritol plus 1 tsp Stevia Glycerite

1/3 cup Blanched almond flour

1 tsp ground cinnamon

1/4 cup butter, softened

Preheat oven to 375 degrees F. Prepare pie shell, by beating all
ingredients together. Pat into a pie pan (using fingers), then place in oven
to bake for 12 minutes. Meanwhile, beat sweetener, cream cheese, eggs
and 2 tablespoons flaxseeds in a large mixing bowl until smooth. Stir in
vanilla and salt. Fold in rhubarb. Pour rhubarb mixture into pie shell.
Bake for 30 minutes in the preheated oven. Meanwhile, combine
sweetener, 1/3 cup Blanched almond flour, and cinnamon in a small
bowl. Cut in butter with fork or pastry blender until mixture resembles
coarse crumbs. Set aside. Remove pie from oven. Reduce oven
temperature to 350 degrees F. Sprinkle topping mixture evenly over pie.
Return pie to oven and bake until filling is set and crust and topping are
golden brown, about 30 minutes.

RHUBARB CRISP

1 cup Erythritol plus 2 tsp Stevia
Glycerite
1 8 oz. package cream cheese
2 eggs
1/2 tsp vanilla extract
1/4 tsp Celtic sea salt
3 cups chopped fresh rhubarb
(option: Sub 1 cup rhubarb for a
low sugar berry like strawberries)
Topping:
1/3 cup Erythritol plus 1 tsp Stevia Glycerite
1/3 cup Crushed almonds/pecans/walnuts
1/3 cup flaxseed meal
1 tsp ground cinnamon
1/4 cup butter, softened

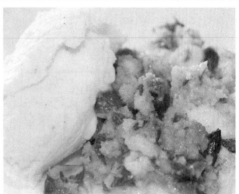

Preheat oven to 375 degrees F. Beat sweetener, cream cheese, eggs in a
large mixing bowl until smooth. Stir in vanilla and salt. Fold in rhubarb.
Pour rhubarb mixture into casserole dish. Bake for 30 minutes in the
preheated oven. Meanwhile, combine 1/3 cup Erythritol, 1/3 cup
crushed nuts, flaxseeds and cinnamon in a small bowl. Cut in butter with
fork or pastry blender until mixture resembles coarse crumbs. Set aside.
Remove rhubarb mixture from oven. Reduce oven temperature to 350
degrees F. Sprinkle topping mixture evenly over pie. Return crisp to oven
and bake until filling is set and crust and topping are golden brown,
about 30 minutes. Serves 8.

NUTRITIONAL INFO (per serving) = 235 calories, 5.5g carbs, 3g fiber

ZUCCHINI CRISP

8 cups cubed peeled zucchini
1/4 cup lemon juice
1/4 cup Erythritol and 1 tsp Stevia Glycerite
2 tsp ground cinnamon
1 tsp ground nutmeg
Topping:
3/4 cup Erythritol and 1 tsp Stevia Glycerite
1 cup chopped pecans
1 cup almond flour
2/3 cup cold butter

In a bowl, combine the zucchini, lemon juice, sweetener, cinnamon and nutmeg; mix well. Pour into a greased 13-in. x 9-in. x 2-in. baking dish.

For topping, combine sweetener, pecans and almond flour in a bowl; cut in butter until crumbly. Sprinkle over the zucchini mixture. Bake at 375 degrees F for 45-50 minutes or until bubbly and the zucchini is tender.

NUTRITIONAL COMPARISON per cup:
Apple = 95 calories, 21 carbs, 4 fiber
Zucchini = 20 calories, 4 carbs, 1 fiber

CONSULTATION SERVICES

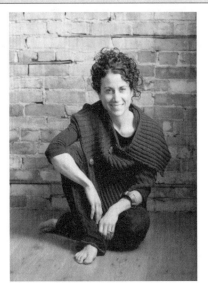

Contact Maria Emmerich at:
WWW.MARIANUTRITION.COM
WWW.MARIAHEALTH.BLOGSPOT.COM